Now What?

A Patient's Guide to Recovery after Mastectomy

About the Authors

Amy Curran Baker, MA, OTR/L, has over fourteen years of experience as an Occupational Therapist, including treating adult populations throughout all stages of post-surgical recovery. Ms. Baker became interested in mastectomy/reconstruction care in 2008 after helping her sister Linda recover from a prophylactic mastectomy. Less than two months later, Ms. Baker was diagnosed with breast cancer herself and underwent a mastectomy with reconstruction. Ms. Baker is an active breast cancer awareness advocate, having participated in print and media interviews on the subject of hereditary breast cancer and reconstruction options. Ms. Baker is a graduate of Smith College and New York University. She lives in the Greater New York City area with her husband and two daughters.

MaryBeth Curran Brown, RN, is a veteran nurse with nearly twenty years of experience. MaryBeth's professional interests include traveling home care nursing, oncology/infusion therapy, and rural home health nursing care. She lives and works in rural Maine.

Linda Curran, MSN, APRN, has practiced for nine years as a Board-certified Advanced Practice Registered Nurse specializing in women's health. Linda's professional interests include breast cancer screening and prevention, *BRCA*, and other hereditary cancer syndromes. Linda has published in the nursing journal *Lifelines* and is employed at a community health clinic in West Oahu, Hawaii. Linda underwent a bilateral prophylactic mastectomy with reconstruction in 2008. She lives in Hawaii with her husband and two children.

Now What?
A Patient's Guide to Recovery after Mastectomy

Amy Curran Baker, MA, OTR/L

With
MaryBeth Curran Brown, RN
and
Linda Curran, MSN, APRN

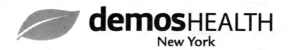

demosHEALTH
New York

Visit our website at www.demoshealth.com

ISBN: 978-1-9363-0325-0
ebook ISBN: 978-1-6170-5101-2

Acquisitions Editor: Noreen Henson
Compositor: Techset

Medical information provided by Demos Health, in the absence of a visit with a healthcare professional, must be considered as an educational service only. This book is not designed to replace a physician's independent judgment about the appropriateness or risks of a procedure of therapy for a given patient. Our purpose is to provide you with information that will help you make your own healthcare decisions.

The information and opinions provided here are believed to be accurate and sound, based on the best judgment available to the authors, editors, and publisher, but readers who fail to consult appropriate health authorities assume the risk of injuries. The publisher is not responsible for errors or omissions. The editors and publisher welcome any reader to report to the publisher any discrepancies or inaccuracies noticed.

CIP data is available from the Library of Congress.

Special discounts on bulk quantities of Demos Health books are available to corporations, professional associations, pharmaceutical companies, healthcare organizations, and other qualifying groups. For details, please contact:

Special Sales Department
Demos Medical Publishing
11 West 42nd Street, 15th Floor
New York, NY 10036
Phone: 800-532-8663 or 212-683-0072
Fax: 212-941-7842
E-mail: specialsales@demosmedical.com

Printed in the United States of America by Gasch Printing.
14 / 5 4 3 2

In memory of
Aunt Ruth and Aunt Joan

For Eric, Phoebe, and Claire Bear

Contents

Foreword

Breast cancer remains a prevalent disease in the United States with approximately 240,000 cases diagnosed each year. It remains the most common form of cancer in women and the second leading cause of cancer death in women. Luckily, treatments for breast cancer have improved dramatically over the past two decades. With improved scientific advancements and better directed therapy, we have begun seeing a slow decline in breast cancer mortality since 1998.

Surgery remains a common treatment for all breast cancer patients; even with the advent of breast conserving surgeries (i.e., lumpectomy) in the 1980s, mastectomy remains an important surgical treatment for patients. There has even been an increase in the use of mastectomy during the past ten years due to improved surgical techniques such as skin sparing and nipple sparing procedures, as well as improved reconstructive options such as muscle preserving DIEP flaps and direct-to-implant reconstructions. The increased use of risk reduction or prophylactic mastectomies for high-risk women has also become increasingly more frequent since we have found one of the genetic links to both breast and ovarian cancers (*BRCA* genes). For these reasons, it has become even more important that a book such as this, a resource guide for women undergoing mastectomy, be available.

We can tell you that, as surgeons specializing in breast surgery and reconstruction, we always receive questions from patients both before and after mastectomy regarding their limitations, recovery time, exercise routines, pain control, and after care. Given the ever-expanding amount of knowledge doctors have obtained in the treatment of breast cancer, we as physicians have found it more difficult to condense our discussions into easily understood presentations that can be fully grasped by all patients. The use of visual

tools has been very helpful but still does not portray the full psychological or physical impact from the surgery, which can be very variable depending upon the individual patient. To guide patients
through these variable aspects of breast cancer surgical treatment
and recovery, Amy Curran Baker and her sisters MaryBeth and
Linda have created a really great resource for patients that will
help patients both before and after surgery and significantly aid in
their recoveries. And who better than two nurses and an occupational therapist, two of whom have themselves experienced mastectomies, to help patients learn from their own stories of recovery.

The authors have addressed both the psychological and physical
aspects of mastectomy and also the reconstructive process. They
write the book from a patient's perspective, adding personal
stories as well as expert occupational therapy advice, which are
often not well covered by physicians in their zeal to help the
patient understand all the factual medical information. In an age
where information is so readily available through electronic
sources yet is often misunderstood or even misinterpreted, it is
refreshing to see a well-written resource that condenses factually
referenced information into a form that a patient can understand
and continually refer to for advice.

Andrew Ashikari, MD, FACS
Assistant Professor of Surgery
New York Medical College
Co-Director Ashikari Breast Center
St. John's Riverside Healthcare System and
Hudson Valley Hospital Center

Andrew Salzberg, MD
Professor of Surgery and Chief of Plastic Surgery
New York Medical College
New York Group for Plastic Surgery

Introduction

This year thousands of women in the United States diagnosed with breast cancer will undergo mastectomy. Many more will choose to undergo prophylactic mastectomy because they have a significant risk of developing breast cancer at some point in their lifetimes.

In 2008, I was one of these women. At age 39, I was diagnosed with invasive ductal cancer. I opted for bilateral mastectomy with direct to implant reconstruction. I have two children, a busy life, and a long family history of breast cancer. I knew what I wanted to do and I couldn't wait to do it.

Within one month of being diagnosed I had my mastectomy and was on the road to recovery. But after the surgery I had a lot of questions: What about these drains? Why am I so tired all the time? Should I worry about lymphedema? As an occupational therapist who is trained to help people become as independent as possible in the face of a variety of disabilities and post-surgical conditions, I knew some of the answers from my own clinical training and experience. But a surprising amount of information came from speaking with other women who had gone through what I was going through, visiting on-line message boards, and when I couldn t find the answers – just plain winging it. I remember wishing there was a book, a resource for all of the information I needed. Nothing fancy, just the basics ...

So three years later – and feeling better than ever – I decided to create such a resource. I have enlisted two of my sisters, MaryBeth, a seasoned registered nurse, and Linda, a women's health nurse practitioner and mastectomy patient herself, to help me with some of the nursing-oriented topics. We have included information on the key issues that post-mastectomy and reconstruction patients will encounter and need to know about: preparing for surgery, what to expect when you awake after surgery, the first few days in the hospital, drain management, dressing and bathing, scar massage, lymphedema prevention, and more. We have compiled all of these topics together into this easy-to-read volume.

If you are reading this book, chances are that you or someone you know is considering mastectomy. Much of what you will read here will apply to all mastectomy patients, whether choosing to undergo reconstruction or not. Everyone's experience will differ slightly depending upon individual choices and circumstances. With this in mind, I have shared my own mastectomy experience and I have enlisted the help of over 50 other mastectomy "veterans" who have responded to surveys about their own mastectomy and reconstruction experiences. They have all graciously agreed to share their advice and stories with you. Perhaps you will relate to their experiences in a way that will help you feel less alone during a very daunting and overwhelming process.

I hope that surgical oncologists and plastic surgeons will share this book with their mastectomy patients at a pre-operative visit so that their patients can refer to it throughout the process of preparing for and recovering from mastectomy. And once its usefulness has ceased, I hope that patients will pass it along to friends and family members who may be preparing for their own journey through mastectomy.

Amy Curran Baker

Acknowledgments

There are a great many people who have had a hand in creating this book and ushering it through to completion. First and foremost, I want to thank the women of FORCE and Support Connection. They are the mastectomy "veterans" who responded to our surveys, offered their advice for recovery, and generously shared their mastectomy experiences and stories so that – going forward – other women would have the answers they need. Thanks in particular to Sue Friedman, DVM, Executive Director of Facing Our Risk of Cancer Empowered, for allowing access to the FORCE message boards and for creating such a wonderful support community in FORCE.

I would also like to thank Sara Cohen, OTR/L, CLT-LANA, Memorial Sloan-Kettering Cancer Center. Sara offered her expertise and contributions for the Lymphedema Prevention section and provided much needed answers for the Rehabilitation After Breast Surgery section of the book. Thanks also to Holly Cline and Kim Dell of Amoena International for providing input on the Breast Prosthesis portion of the book. Thanks to Heidi Moncrief and Gabriel Rudow of Healthwise, Inc., for providing the breast reconstruction medical illustrations. Thanks also to the organizations that allowed permission for important mastectomy related information to be reprinted including: The American Cancer Society, The National Lymphedema Network, UCSF Breast Care Center Website, and The American Board for Certification in Orthotics, Prosthetics, and Pedorthics.

Other friends, colleagues, and physicians who reviewed the book, offered comments and expertise, and cheered me on along the way include Sharon Smith, MA, OTR/L, S. Lynn Karidis, PT, owner of Breast Cancer Rehabilitation of Westchester, and Tina Coyle, MS, NCC, LPC, Peer Counselor, Support Connection. Also, I would like to thank my fabulous medical team including Andrew Ashikari, MD, C. Andrew Salzberg, MD, and Elizabeth Chabner Thompson, MD, MPH, all talented physicians and genuinely kind, caring individuals who offered their feedback and medical expertise in reviewing the manuscript.

Thanks to Noreen Henson, Editor at Demos Health, for believing that this project was important and recognizing that it would ultimately help many women faced with the prospect of mastectomy. My appreciation also goes to Joanne Jay and Tom Hastings at Demos for their tireless efforts in bringing *Now What?* to completion.

Thanks to my sisters and co-authors, MaryBeth Curran Brown and Linda Curran, for the their ongoing contributions, editing, reviewing, expertise, encouragement, and putting up with me! Finally, thank you to all of the members of my family, including my parents Thomas and Nancy Curran, my "big" sisters MaryBeth, Jennifer, and Linda, my in-laws Nancy and Ralph Baker, my husband Eric, and my daughters Phoebe and Claire for their love, support, and patience these many months.

1

Making the Difficult Decisions

If you are considering a mastectomy because you have been diagnosed with breast cancer or you are contemplating *prophylactic mastectomy* due to heightened hereditary risk, you have come to the right source. This book is about planning for and recovering from mastectomy. If you are in the early stages of decision making and haven't yet decided about having a mastectomy, you should know that there are some wonderful resources out there to help guide you through your decision-making process. There is an extensive resource section at the back of this book to help with this decision. Note that much of the planning and recovery from your mastectomy procedure is related to the type of procedure that you ultimately select.

My Story

Each of us has her own reason for making the decision to have a mastectomy. For some women, mastectomy is one of several possible treatment options. For others, mastectomy may be the only option. Overall, however, my situation and decision-making process may have been a little different than most. I was 39 years old with two kids and a significant family history of breast cancer. My mother, my maternal grandmother, and my maternal Aunt Ruth had all been diagnosed. My mother had been diagnosed in her 50s, my grandmother in her 80s, and my Aunt Ruth in her late 30s. And here I was,

1

almost 40 years old and I had only been for one mammogram so far. What I know now is that with my family history, I should have been getting a yearly mammogram and twice yearly breast exams beginning at age 35. I had my first mammogram at age 32 when I thought I felt a lump. My wonderful OB/GYN at the time, who had seen me through the birth of my first child, felt it too, and another lump besides. She immediately sent me for a mammogram that, thankfully, came back normal.

So there I was seven years later. Life was busy and I was in the trenches of parenting two wonderfully spirited young girls. I was muddling along, in full denial of the fact that I have a real risk of breast cancer and should go for another mammogram. Actually, I wasn't in *full* denial. I had made several appointments — and I had canceled several appointments. Once I even actually showed up for my appointment only to be turned away because I didn't have the necessary referral. I did a monthly self-exam in the shower but sometimes I didn't really know what I was feeling. Looking back I may have felt a lump in my right breast but I was never exactly sure what I was feeling so I didn't pursue it — a bump here, a rib there. What was cancer going to feel like anyway?

So when my sister Linda springs it on me in late January of 2008 that she is planning on coming east from her home in Hawaii to undergo a *bilateral prophylactic mastectomy*, my jaw drops. But I try not to let her see my reaction because I want her to feel supported in what, undoubtedly, has to be one of the hardest decisions any person can make. To take essentially healthy breasts and opt to remove them — and in the process causing yourself pain, discomfort, and inconvenience — in order to reduce the risk of developing cancer down the line was, I felt, a decision that really took some guts.

Linda had a history of *atypical ductal hyperplasia*, which basically means that there were some unusual cells growing in the milk ducts of her breasts. They weren't cancerous cells but they weren't typical cells either. Her physician and a *genetic counselor* had cautioned her that she had a significant risk, based on this diagnosis and family history, of developing breast cancer "at some point" in her lifetime.

Linda had it all planned out. She had done the research and found a small hospital that was doing really cutting-edge work in the areas of mastectomy and breast reconstruction. Coincidentally, the hospital just happened to be about 30 minutes from my house in New York. So she would fly from Hawaii with her husband and baby daughter, have the surgery, and then come to my house to recuperate for two weeks or so afterward.

I sat in the waiting room with Mike, Linda's husband, and held their beautiful seven-month-old baby girl while Linda underwent a bilateral prophylactic mastectomy with *direct to implant reconstruction*, popularly known as *one-step surgery*. The surgery went beautifully and her physicians, a surgical oncologist and a plastic surgeon, met us in the waiting room with broad smiles and positive reports — the initial *pathology* was all clear; that is, no cancer had been found.

Two days later Linda was discharged from the hospital. But before we left the hospital, I decided that the least I could do was go to the breast center and set myself up for a mammogram. I mean, look at how proactive Linda was being and here I was burying my head in the sand still. So I booked it.

Linda's recovery went well. Two days after discharge, drains and bandages neatly concealed, she was feeling well enough to enjoy Super Bowl Sunday at a local hotel bar while sipping on a Shirley Temple. Nine days after surgery she flew home to Hawaii with a new-found peace of mind.

And that is where my story really picks up. In late February I went for that mammogram. I was nervous as hell. They took the pictures and then told me to wait for the results. I waited a long time before they finally sent me home but I was nervous because I had a feeling something was wrong. That night my primary care physician called me to say that they found something and they wanted me to come back for additional views. "What we might be looking at here is *invasive ductal cancer*," she said. I'm pretty sure that I almost died right then. I went back the next morning and the mammogram technician took additional images. The radiologist called me in and showed me the picture of my right breast blown up to the size of my head. There were some red pen marks circling the "problem" areas.

I don't think I ate or slept much for the next few weeks. I did cry a lot, though. I allowed myself only once to go "there." You know the place. The place where I am not here to take care of my two girls, who at the time were ages three and eight. I was seen a week or so later by my sister's surgical oncologist, now *my* surgical oncologist, too. I almost passed out in the examination room when he told me that, given my family history, he thought there was at least a 50:50 chance that this was cancer. Looking back now, I think he was being careful with his estimate, probably in an effort to help me keep it together enough to make it through that appointment. I have since learned that when you have a mammogram, your radiologist assigns something called a *BI-RADS* score to your images. BI-RADS stands for *Breast Imaging-Reporting and Data Systems*,[1] it is a rating scale of 1 to 6. Each number corresponds with a description of what has been found on a mammogram. A number 1 means the mammogram is all clear for cancer. A number 6 means that your cancer has already been confirmed by biopsy and now they are just imaging it for treatment purposes. I earned a BI-RADS score of 5, which meant that there was about a 95 percent chance that my mammogram was positive for breast cancer.

My physician referred me to an affiliated hospital for a *biopsy*. The results came back as *DCIS (ductal carcinoma in situ)* Stage 0 cancer. I was both shocked and elated — shocked that at age 39 I would be diagnosed with breast cancer of any kind; elated that, after weeks of worrying, my cancer was found to be Stage 0, which meant that it hadn't spread beyond the milk ducts into the surrounding breast tissue. Maybe I had gotten lucky.

And that's where this book comes in. I quickly decided that I, too, would undergo a bilateral mastectomy with immediate reconstruction. I was lucky because Linda's experience had not only prompted me to act but also paved the way for me.

Honestly, I didn't really think, I just acted. I had met the surgeons, been to the hospital, and knew enough about the process to anticipate what my recovery would be like. And once I had locked into a plan it made me crazy to have people trying to talk me out of it — they always seemed to be pushing for me to get a *lumpectomy*, which is when the surgeon removes just the cancer and a bit of the normal surrounding tissue from your breast. Lumpectomies are a good option because they allow the surgeon to preserve the breast to the greatest extent possible. But I wanted a mastectomy, that much I knew for sure. I had spoken at length with my physicians about the decision I was making and I wanted some reassurance that my hereditary lot in life was not going to sneak up on me again and catch me by surprise when I least expected it.

I decided that my left breast, the non-cancerous breast, would undergo a *prophylactic skin sparing, nipple-sparing mastectomy* with *direct to implant reconstruction*. That's a lot of fancy lingo for: They saved the nipple and the skin covering my breast but they took out the breast tissue and inserted an implant under my *pectoralis major* muscle. Because I didn't have cancer on that side, this surgery was considered "prophylactic"; in other words, it was an opportunity to head off cancer from developing in that area in the future. There are many reasons for having the surgery done bilaterally (on both sides). Besides the obvious health reason I just mentioned, it is also easier for a plastic surgeon to achieve symmetry of the breasts if both sides are being reconstructed.

My right breast, the cancer side, underwent a skin-sparing mastectomy with the same type of implant reconstruction. They kept most of my skin so it was considered "skin sparing" but my surgeon felt that the cancer was too close to the nipple to be safe. So the nipple would not be spared. I didn't mind. Later on, several months after I had healed from my initial surgery, my plastic surgeon would fashion a nipple for me through some sort of origami-like technique using my own skin and the surrounding scar tissue. Finally, they would finish the job with a tattoo that would leave me with a reasonable facsimile of a real nipple.

I remember the frustration I felt at not having the mastectomy sooner. I wanted to fast track the whole thing. I wanted those things off yesterday. But I would have to settle for having the surgery a month or so after my diagnosis on April 16, 2008. I knew that the recovery process was not simple but it wasn't awful either. I had watched my sister's recovery and I was a rehabilitation professional myself, so I had those things going for me. But I still felt there was a lot of information I just didn't know. I turned to the Facing our Risk of Cancer Empowered (FORCE) on-line message boards on a daily basis. FORCE is a non-profit organization devoted to providing support to women with increased familial risk for breast and ovarian cancer. Many of these women have tested positive for the *BRCA 1* or *2* genes. People who are *BRCA 1* or *2* positive carry a gene that puts them at significantly increased risk for breast and ovarian cancer. I tested "negative" for the *BRCA* gene but, as my physician explained to me, there is a whole population of women like me out there who have strong family histories of breast cancer yet test *BRCA* negative. This may simply be because we carry a gene mutation that researchers haven't discovered yet. The women posting on the FORCE board were an excellent source of information about hereditary breast cancer, options available for *surveillance* and treatment, and various post-mastectomy recovery issues. And they were so supportive that I couldn't help but feel at home there.

When I went back for my pathology results a week after the surgery, I was surprised to learn that my breast cancer *had* been invasive. Although the small biopsied area had only shown DCIS or Stage 0 cancer, there was also a small area of invasive cancer as well as other areas of DCIS and cancer extending into the *lobules*. So in the end, I would undergo *adjuvant chemotherapy*. The chemotherapy, along with my mastectomy, and later the oral medication *tamoxifen*, would give me the added insurance I needed that my cancer wasn't coming back. And as far as I was concerned, the mastectomy had been the best choice for me and the pathology results confirmed it. I was happy with how I looked reconstruction-wise and I hadn't really had too much pain. Discomfort, yes, but full on pain, not so much of that really. And now I could rest easy that the cancer was gone and if I could just get over this next chemotherapy hurdle, life would go back to normal. And it did.

Surgical Options

My story complete, that bring us back to the whole decision-making process. Let's begin with the surgical options. In the next few pages, I will provide a basic overview of the different types of breast surgery that your physician may recommend if you have been diagnosed with breast cancer or are considering prophylactic mastectomy. I will also review some of the reconstructive options that may be available to you. This is not an exhaustive list; for the most in-depth information on this topic, see Kathy Steligo's classic, *The Breast Reconstruction Guidebook*, listed in the resources section at the back of this book. Her book is widely considered to be the most thorough resource on the topic of breast reconstruction options.

If you have been diagnosed with breast cancer, your surgeon may tell you that you have the option to have either a lumpectomy or a mastectomy. Here are some basics about each type of surgery.

Lumpectomy

With a lumpectomy, the surgeon removes the cancerous tumor and a small amount of healthy surrounding tissue. This surrounding tissue is referred to as the *margin*. Surgeons want to be sure that they get good or "clean" margins because then they can be reasonably assured that they have removed all of the cancerous tissue from the breast. The *nipple and areolar complex (NAC)* is typically not removed with this type of surgery. Usually *radiation therapy* is also prescribed as part of the treatment after lumpectomy. Lumpectomy is considered a *breast conserving surgery* because it allows the patient to keep most of her breast and there is typically less cosmetic impact. If margins are found to be positive after surgery, a *re-excision* may be required in order to remove all of the remaining cancer.[2]

Mastectomy

If your surgeon advises that you are a candidate for mastectomy, you should be aware that there are several different types of mastectomy. Each type differs based on the amount of tissue that needs to be removed from the breast and the surrounding areas. Your breast surgeon will make a recommendation about what procedure is best for you based on your unique health circumstances. The different types of mastectomy are as follows:

- **Simple Mastectomy:** With this procedure the breast tissue and the NAC are removed but the underlying chest muscles and the axillary lymph nodes are left intact. This procedure is also called a *total mastectomy*.[3]
- **Modified Radical Mastectomy:** This procedure involves removing all of the breast tissue, the nipple areolar complex, and the lower axillary lymph nodes.[4]

- **Skin Sparing Mastectomy:** This type of surgery removes the breast tissue but leaves most of the skin over the breast intact. The nipple and areola are also removed.
- **Nipple Sparing Mastectomy:** With this procedure the underlying breast tissue is removed; however, the skin and nipple/areolar complex are preserved.
- **Prophylactic Mastectomy:** This is when a patient undergoes mastectomy prior to receiving a cancer diagnosis. The procedure is a preventive or risk-reducing measure based on individual medical history, family history, or *BRCA* status.
- **Radical Mastectomy:** The entire breast is removed as well as the skin, nipple, some or all of the underlying muscle tissue, and all of the axillary lymph nodes. This procedure is no longer performed as often as it once was due to advances in mastectomy technique and breast conserving surgeries.[5]

There are many variables for what makes each of us good candidates for one type of surgery over another. A nipple sparing mastectomy, for instance, is unlikely to be recommended if the cancerous tumor is large or located within two centimeters of the nipple. It also may not be recommended for women who are very large breasted or who have significant sagging of the breasts, also known as *ptosis*. A radical mastectomy may be the best choice when the tumor is large and the cancer has spread to the chest wall. Consult with your breast surgeon about what type of procedure is recommended for you.

Lymph Node Removal

As well as surgical options, there should also be a discussion with your physician about lymph nodes. *Lymph nodes* are the small, bean-like structures that pick up and move lymph fluid through our bodies, returning it to the blood stream. Lymph is made up of water, bacteria, fat, and parts of white and red blood cells.[6] If you have been diagnosed with breast cancer, whether or not the cancer has spread to your lymph nodes will help determine the *staging* of your cancer. *Axillary lymph node dissection (ALND)*, or removal of all or some of the lymph nodes in the underarm area, used to be routine practice when a woman was having a mastectomy. Today, techniques have improved and are significantly less invasive. Your surgeon will most likely recommend a *sentinel lymph node biopsy (SLNB)* to determine if the cancer has progressed to your lymph nodes. In September of 2010, the National Surgical Adjuvant Breast and Bowel Project released a study confirming that women who underwent sentinel lymph node biopsy had the same survival rates after eight years as the women who underwent axillary lymph node dissection.[7]

Sentinel Lymph Node Mapping and Biopsy

The *sentinel lymph node* is the node that the lymph fluid first encounters when exiting the affected breast. This node acts like a sentinel or "guard," allowing fluid to pass to the other lymph nodes. There can be more than one sentinel node found and on average about two nodes are typically found. Through a process called *sentinel lymph node mapping* or *lymphoscintigraphy*, a radiologist or surgeon is able to determine the location of the sentinel lymph node(s). In this procedure, a radioisotope and/or blue dye is injected into the affected breast. The radiologist, during the lymphoscintigraphy, injects the radioisotope to determine the location of the sentinel lymph node(s) and marks it on the skin for the breast surgeon. The surgeon uses a gamma counter to identify the radioactive tracer during the surgery, thus identifying the first draining lymph node(s) of the breast. During the surgery, the surgeon may also inject a blue dye into the breast, which also drains into the sentinel node(s) and further enhances the identification of the sentinel node(s) by turning then blue. In these ways, the sentinel node(s) can be removed and checked for cancer. A sentinel lymph node biopsy is not usually recommended for prophylactic surgeries; however, some physicians will recommend it for women with a known genetic mutation. If the sentinel lymph node is cancer free, the reasonable assumption can be made that the next lymph nodes in the sequential chain will also be cancer free.[8] This eliminates the need for removing more lymph nodes than absolutely necessary. A condition called *lymphedema* — a condition that occurs when a person's lymphatic system does not drain lymph fluid properly — can occur when lymph nodes are removed, injured, or radiated so it is preferable to leave as many healthy lymph nodes intact as possible. After breast surgery with removal of lymph nodes, lymphedema can occur in the arm and/or chest area and, because the lymph channels are altered, can cause swelling in those areas. It should be noted that sometimes lymph nodes tend to be in close proximity to each other so even though you may be having a sentinel lymph node biopsy, it is possible that more than one lymph node will be removed with this process.

Axillary Lymph Node Dissection

If the sentinel lymph node biopsy reveals that cancer is present, an axillary lymph node dissection may be performed. With axillary lymph node dissection there is a greater chance that a person will develop lymphedema; however, this largely depends upon the number of lymph nodes removed. The more lymph nodes removed, the greater the chance of developing lymphedema later on. That said, even with sentinel lymph node biopsy, which presumably only involves one or few lymph nodes, there is a small chance of lymphedema developing. See the section on Rehabilitation Questions and Answers and Lymphedema Prevention for more information about this topic. One important point to note is that once you have already undergone a mastectomy, a sentinel lymph node biopsy is no longer possible. The reason for this is that the tracer dye cannot be injected once the breast tissue has been removed. It makes it important, if there is a suspicion that cancer may have reached the lymph nodes, to take advantage of the sentinel lymph node biopsy at the time of the mastectomy in order to avoid axillary lymph node dissection at a later date.

Reconstruction Options

The next question: If you have chosen to have a mastectomy, do you want breast reconstruction? You should know that thanks to The Women's Health and Cancer Rights Act of 1998 (WHCRA), health insurers that cover mastectomy must also offer coverage for reconstructive services and certain post-operative complications.[9] Under WHCRA, a patient who has undergone a mastectomy is entitled to reconstruction of *both* the affected and unaffected breasts in an effort to create a balanced and natural appearance of the breasts. Prosthetic breast forms, lymphedema treatment, and treatment for other post-operative complications must also be covered under this law. The United States Department of Labor and the American Cancer Society websites, which are listed in the Resources section of this book, both contain lots of information about WHCRA and include lists of frequently asked questions that may be helpful.

I'm proud to say that my home state of New York has taken this issue one step further and recently passed legislation that requires physicians to tell patients about their reconstructive options before performing any surgeries to remove cancer.[10] The purpose of this law is to help women make informed choices about mastectomy, lumpectomy, and the various types of reconstruction that are available to them. When women are given this information early in the process, they are then likely to have all the necessary tools to make the most informed decisions they can about the options available. Hopefully other states will follow New York's lead and adopt similar legislation in the future.

Most physicians' offices will have a person on staff whose job it is to negotiate with your health insurance company to get your surgical procedure covered. If you decide that you want a specific type of procedure that is not covered within your network, you can apply for something called a "gap in coverage exception." With adequate documentation from your physician, you may be successful in getting your insurance company to cover your procedure of choice.

To Reconstruct or Not to Reconstruct?

Sometimes women choose to have no breast reconstruction. Other times, women want or need to delay their breast reconstruction surgery. This may be the case if the woman has a long treatment road ahead of her consisting of radiation or chemotherapy, or if she wants to take it slow and examine all the options before making a decision about what type of reconstruction to pursue. Getting a breast cancer diagnosis in itself is such an overwhelming event that having to make a lot of decisions about reconstruction may be too much all at once. When I was diagnosed I didn't know the first thing about breast reconstruction. If I hadn't had the benefit of my sister's experience, I probably would have chosen to delay my breast reconstruction to give myself a chance to explore all of the available options.

Implant and Flap Overview

If you ultimately decide on breast reconstruction, what type do you prefer: reconstruction with implants or reconstruction using your own tissue? When implants are used there are a couple of options: tissue expanders or direct to implant. With both types of surgery, the final result is that an implant is placed under the chest muscle and skin to form the breast mound. With autologous or "flap" procedures, the patient's own tissue is used to form the breast mound. Here is a quick overview of some of the most frequently performed types of breast reconstruction as outlined by the American Cancer Society.[11]

Implant Options

Direct to Implant or One-Stage Immediate Breast Reconstruction

With direct to implant reconstruction both the mastectomy and the reconstruction are done within one surgical procedure. First, the breast tissue is removed by the breast surgeon and then the plastic surgeon takes over to place the implants. The implants are filled with saline or silicone, depending upon the type you and your surgeon have agreed upon ahead of time. Because there usually isn't enough muscle tissue to cover the implant immediately, a *tissue matrix* like Alloderm™ may be used to form a pocket to hold the implant in place. The tissue matrix provides a foundation for your own tissue to grow. It acts something like scaffolding, covering the muscle and keeping the implant in place until your own tissue has grown enough to cover the area. This is a fairly new type of surgery that is gaining popularity because it is a relatively brief surgical procedure and recovery time tends to be short. Not every person is a candidate for this type of surgery, so check with your plastic surgeon about your specific situation.

Tissue Expander to Implant or Two-Stage Reconstruction

This is the traditional form of implant surgery. With this type of surgery the breast tissue is removed and then a *tissue expander*, like a balloon, is placed under the chest muscle. Over a period of several months the expander is gradually filled with saline through a small valve until the skin and muscle have stretched adequately and the optimal breast size has been achieved. Later, a second surgery is performed to swap the temporary expander for a more permanent implant.

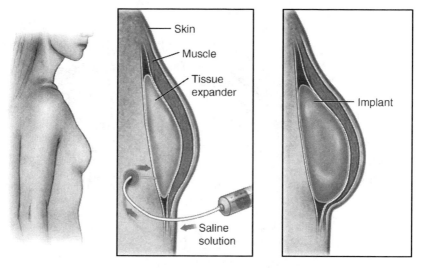

Tissue Expander to Implant (Two-Stage Reconstruction).
Copyright © Healthwise, Inc.

"Flap" or Autologous Tissue Options

With *autologous* or *flap* procedures, the patient's own tissue is used to form the breast mound. Many people who do not want a foreign object such as an implant in their bodies choose this option. Whether or not you are a candidate for this type of surgery may depend upon how much fat or extra tissue you have in various areas of your body. The length of surgery and recovery period for flap procedures is typically longer than for implant surgeries. The American Cancer Society website outlines many of the most common types of flap procedure[12]:

■ With a ***deep inferior epigastric artery perforator flap***, popularly known as a ***DIEP***, the surgeon takes tissue, fat, small blood vessels, and skin from the abdomen and relocates it to the chest to form the breast mound. As with many of the autologous procedures, this is microsurgery and there will be two surgical sites: the donor site from which the tissue is harvested and the reconstructed breast site. Using a special type of microscope, the surgeon reattaches the small blood vessels so that the transplanted tissue is viable. This procedure provides a "tummy tuck" because it removes tissue from the abdomen, just below the bikini line.

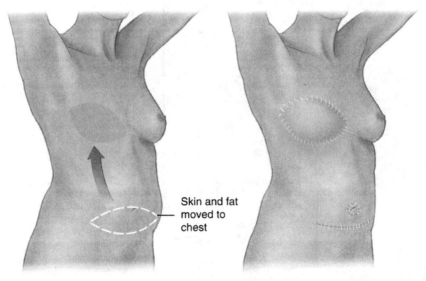

Skin and fat moved to chest

Deep Inferior Epigastric Artery Perforator (DIEP) Flap.
Copyright © Healthwise, Inc.

■ With the **transverse rectus abdominis muscle flap** procedure, also called a **TRAM**, there are two options: the *pedicle TRAM flap* or the *free TRAM flap*. With the pedicle TRAM flap, one of the rectus abdominis muscles of the abdomen is rerouted up under the skin to form the breast mound. The original blood supply is left intact. Mesh may be used to secure the area of the abdomen where the flap has been removed. With a free TRAM flap, the muscle, skin, blood vessels, and fat are removed from the donor site and reattached at the reconstruction site. This again requires the blood vessels to be reattached through microsurgery in order for the transplanted tissue to be viable.

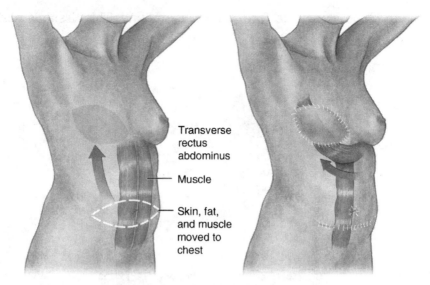

Transverse
rectus
abdominus

Muscle

Skin, fat,
and muscle
moved to
chest

Transverse Rectus Abdominis Muscle (TRAM) Flap.
Copyright © Healthwise, Inc.

■ The **latissimus dorsi flap** is a combination procedure that involves rerouting of the latissimus dorsi muscle of the back to form a pocket on the chest for a breast implant. Sometimes there is enough tissue to form the breast without using an implant.

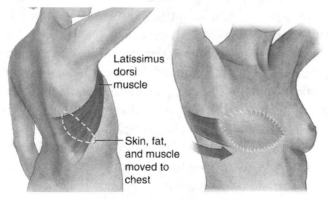

Latissimus
dorsi
muscle

Skin, fat,
and muscle
moved to
chest

Latissimus Dorsi Flap.
Copyright © Healthwise, Inc.

■ With a **superior gluteal artery perforator flap** or **SGAP**, the gluteal muscles of the buttocks are used, along with skin, fat, and blood vessels, to form the breast mound. This tissue is reattached with microsurgery.

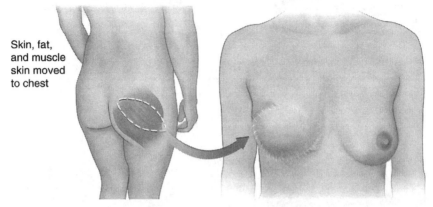

Skin, fat, and muscle skin moved to chest

Superior Gluteal Artery Perforator (SGAP) Flaps.
Copyright © Healthwise, Inc.

Things to Consider

Each of us will want to consider various personal and health issues before making a decision about breast reconstruction. This is an important conversation that should take place between you and your physician. Variables that may impact your reconstruction options include your breast size, amount of ptosis, previously radiated skin, and amount of excess body fat. There are positives and negatives for each type of surgery listed here. For instance, with implants there is a good chance that you will need to have them replaced at some point in your lifetime. The lifespan of today's generation of breast implants is roughly 10–15 years. Also, there continues to be some controversy surrounding the health impact of implants. The U.S. Food and Drug Administration devotes a full section on its website to the safety of breast implants. With autologous procedures, there are two surgical sites to care for and there is always a chance that the flap will not be viable or that there will be residual muscle weakness at the donor site.

I have seen amazing results from both implant and autologous reconstruction. Sometimes the results are so good that you would have difficulty believing that they are not the woman's original breasts. It is important to know your surgeon's level of experience with the procedure you want. Don't be afraid to ask your plastic surgeon for references; there should be former patients who are willing to speak with you and post-operative photos available to review — this is standard in the world of breast reconstruction. The following information has been printed with the permission of the U.S. Food and Drug Administration.

Questions to Ask Your Surgeon about Breast Reconstruction[13]:

You may have additional questions as well.

1. What are all my options for breast reconstruction?
2. What are the risks and complications of each type of breast reconstruction surgery and how common are they?
3. What if my cancer recurs or occurs in the other breast?
4. Will reconstruction interfere with my cancer treatment?
5. How many steps are there in each procedure? What are they? How much experience do you have with each procedure? What is the estimated total cost of each procedure?
6. How long will it take to complete my reconstruction?
7. Do you have before and after photos I can look at for each procedure and what results are reasonable for me?
8. What will my scars look like?
9. What kind of changes in my breast can I expect over time?
10. What kind of changes in my breast can I expect with pregnancy?
11. What are my options if I am dissatisfied with the cosmetic outcome of my breast?
12. How much pain or discomfort will I feel and for how long?
13. How long will I be in the hospital? Will I need blood transfusions, and can I donate my own blood?
14. When will I be able to resume my normal activity (such as athletic activity, sexual activity)?[13]

Choosing Not to Reconstruct

Many women choose not to reconstruct after mastectomy. In fact, it is estimated that 30–40% of women do not reconstruct.[14] Whether this is actually by choice or due to lack of information about the breast reconstruction options available, it represents a significant number of women. As with all of the decisions you will make surrounding mastectomy and breast reconstruction, choosing not to reconstruct is very personal. There are lots of reasons not to reconstruct. Eileen, for example, chose not to reconstruct because:

> *At the time I didn't feel it was important to me. I looked at photos of mastectomies with no reconstruction and I was not bothered by the photos. I wanted the least amount of surgery and the easiest recovery.*

Some women choose not to reconstruct because they want to take time to consider all of their options before rushing into a decision about reconstruction. Others want only one surgery and a quick recovery period so that they can get back to a normal life as soon as possible without having a lot of follow-up restrictions. Other women wait because their breast cancer treatment process is ongoing and may include radiation that can impact reconstruction options. Many women who ultimately opt *not* to undergo breast reconstruction report feelings of freedom and liberation at being "breast free" after mastectomy. And for other women, not having breasts is the end result of failed reconstruction. In this case, going without breasts is not really a choice and can be a devastating development. Regardless of the reason for not reconstructing, there are on-line forums such as Breastfree.org (www.breastfree.org) to support you before and after your mastectomy, and while you adjust to your new body.

Decisions

You should consider consulting with more than one breast surgeon and plastic surgeon before your final decisions about mastectomy and breast reconstruction are made. You should also talk to other patients about their decisions, recovery processes, and cosmetic results. Health insurance issues will also play a role in your decision-making process. Here's some advice from a mastectomy veteran:

Read as much as you can, ask as many questions of the doctors as you can think of. Ask the surgeon to put you in touch with former patients who are willing to talk with you. Get on message boards and communicate with other women who have been there. ALWAYS get a second opinion. Even if there is no doubt about having the surgery, the different perspective of another doctor is very valuable. (Melanie)

As much as possible, take your time, examine your options, and make the decision that feels right for you. Once you feel confident in your decision, don't let people with different opinions throw you off course. Undoubtedly, there will be people — family members, friends, and co-workers — who will not agree with your choice. This can be one of the hardest things to deal with when you are making these tough decisions.

As one who has been down this road, made these incredibly difficult decisions, and gone through this very foreign process myself a few years ago, I want to share with you some of the things I learned that may make your journey through recovery a little easier and, with hope, less frightening. I have also enlisted other mastectomy veterans to share stories of their own recovery experiences in the hope of easing your journey through and beyond mastectomy.

2

Now What?

Getting Ready

By now you have read all of the books, talked to all your friends and family members, and had numerous appointments with doctors. Ideally, you have had long conversations with both your breast surgeon and plastic surgeon about all of the options available to you. Once you have made the decision to move forward with your mastectomy, you will have a lot of preparation to do. There will be pre-operative consultations with your surgeons, pre-operative testing and physicals, insurance companies to deal with, bags to pack, and plans to be made. Here is a good starting point for what to bring when you go to the hospital:

1. This book
2. Loose fitting, elastic waist, silky pajama bottoms
3. Bathrobe
4. Washable slippers
5. Toiletries including flushable wipes and lip balm
6. IPOD and charger, magazines, books
7. Cell phone and charger
8. Earplugs (hospitals can be noisy places)
9. Water bottle with built-in straw

10. Clothing for leaving the hospital. These items should include loose fitting elastic waist pants, underwear, oversized button or zipper front shirt or sweatshirt, slip on shoes.
11. Post-operative bra, *only* if your physician has asked you to purchase it ahead of time.
12. Any necessary paperwork — insurance cards, driver's license, etc. — that may be required at time of admission. Don't bring valuables to the hospital if you can possibly avoid it.

There are many things that you can do to get yourself organized before you go to the hospital. For starters, ask your physicians to write your *post-operative* prescriptions ahead of time. Try to fill the prescriptions in advance so that they are ready when you arrive home from the hospital. Invest in a seven-day pill box organizer; it will help you organize your many medications after surgery. Also, opening those child safety caps is nearly impossible after the surgery, so have the medications already organized in a pill box. Another option is to ask for non-child proof caps to ease opening but be sure to take the necessary precautions if you have young children in the house. Once you have had the surgery, use the chart in the back of this book to keep a running log of your medications.

When I was first discharged from the hospital I went straight home and plopped into bed. I didn't want to be running errands to pick up prescriptions, supplies, or what have you. And I definitely didn't want my husband to be out doing those things because I wanted him home taking care of me! For a while — probably for a few days — I felt more comfortable having someone else around just in case I started to feel sick or something unexpected happened. Happily, nothing ever happened, but I still felt more comfortable knowing there was someone nearby.

If your physician has asked you to buy a specific type of post-operative bra, shop for it ahead of time. Not all physicians will ask you to do this but if they do, the last thing you want to be doing is shopping for bras one or two days after discharge. If you are unsure about what size is best, buy more than one size and return the unused bra after surgery. My Mom and I went to Nordstrom several days before my surgery; she watched the kids while I picked through rack after rack of bras. It was exhausting. I have never been much of a bra shopper, probably because I never *really* needed a bra before. But with my reconstruction, I had the option of going up a cup size or two and I decided to go for it. So I found myself needing a bit more than a tank top with a built in shelf-bra. And my physician happened to have specific recommendations for what type of bra I should buy.

Another thing that you may want to do is ask your physician about surgical restrictions ahead of time and, to the extent possible, organize your home with these restrictions in mind in preparation for your discharge. For example, if lifting a gallon jug of milk is going to mean breaking your lifting restrictions after surgery, buy milk in smaller containers or divide the gallon jug into smaller sized containers ahead of time. Buy easy-to-prepare foods or pre-cook several meals and freeze them ahead of time. One of our mastectomy veterans offers some suggestions here:

> *In preparation for surgery, I paid attention to my usual activities for a couple of weeks, imagining myself with post-op restrictions, made lists, then stocked up on non-perishable supplies, bought smaller/lightweight packages of some things (dog food, laundry detergent) and put things I would need on a regular basis in low cupboards, so I wouldn't have to climb on a stool when I couldn't raise my arms. Best tip, if you can manage it: have someone else do everything! (Jill)*

This is a great blueprint for how to be proactive about your post-operative restrictions. It is much easier to deal with your limitations if you know what they are going to be ahead of time and can plan accordingly. This may include enlisting the help of friends and family for those activities that are going to be impossible to manage without help when you get home. Certain aspects of child care and dog walking come to mind here. You will not be able to lift small children when you get home, so try to line up family members, friends, and babysitters ahead of time to help out. In terms of pet care, very small dogs might not be a problem but walking a larger dog that tends to pull on the leash — as both of my dogs do — is a definite "no no" after surgery. Skip ahead to the home management and child-care sections of this chapter for more ideas about managing these aspects of your life after your mastectomy.

If you are on regular medications like blood thinners, aspirin, or ibuprofen, these medications may need to be stopped prior to surgery under the guidance of your physician. These drugs interfere with blood clotting so they are often avoided for a period before and after your surgery. Ask about this at a pre-operative visit and try to get a time frame for when you can expect to be able to return to your regular medications after surgery. Do not make any changes to your regular medication routines without first consulting your physician.

Getting in and out of bed can be a big challenge after a mastectomy so spend some time thinking about this and experimenting ahead of time. Start by practicing getting in and out of bed without using your arms. Now imagine that your chest and abdominal muscles are sore. Practice *bed mobility* ahead of time so that you are familiar and comfortable with the technique. Review the bed mobility and sleeping sections of this chapter to find out what has worked for other women.

Finally, to the extent possible, plan out and set up your at-home recovery area in advance so that you have easy access to everything you will need. Books, television remote, medications, bottles of water, should be within arm's reach. And you will need lots of pillows to position yourself comfortably.

> *I ... kept a small basket with water, easy-to-open snacks, telephone, television remote next to my chair, and I could easily take it around the house with me if I wanted. (E.)*

The night before or the morning of your surgery, you may be asked to shower with antibacterial soap. Take extra care in washing the breast area in preparation for your surgery. This will help reduce your risk of infection later on.

Getting Ready Review

- Obtain post-operative prescriptions ahead of time.
- Buy post-operative bra ahead of time (if required).
- Get a list of post-operative restrictions and organize your home with these restrictions in mind.

- Talk to your physician about any medications you are taking that may impact blood clotting.
- Practice bed mobility techniques.
- Plan and set-up your at-home recovery area.
- Shower with antibacterial soap the night before your surgery.

Getting ready emotionally is the hardest part of preparing for mastectomy. Again, everyone's situation is different and a lot will depend upon your status going into the surgery: Did you have a cancer diagnosis or are you a *"previvor"*? Previvors are the folks, like my sister Linda, who are survivors of a hereditary predisposition to cancer. They haven't received a cancer diagnosis but may undergo prophylactic mastectomy because they are at high risk for develop- ing breast cancer in the future. I already had breast cancer so I was anxious to get the mastectomy over and done with, and I didn't spend a lot of time thinking about or romanticizing my breasts. When I had cancer I felt like I was on a treadmill. And every single appointment, test, or procedure was getting me closer to my goal: to be cancer free. When I was on that treadmill I didn't look side to side, only straight ahead. For me, that meant not really allowing myself to dwell on what I was "losing," only what I would ultimately gain, which was good health and peace of mind. There is a great T-shirt that says, "Yes, they are fake. My real ones tried to kill me" and that pretty much sums up my feelings going into my mas- tectomy. That's not to say that I didn't have moments of sadness — of course I did. The night before my surgery while I was taking a shower I looked down at my breasts and realized that they would never look this way again. Not that they were ever anything to write home about, mind you. But they were mine; I had breastfed both of my children with these breasts. That was a sad moment but in the end, the relief I felt after the surgery ultimately outweighed my sadness. This was my experience; these were my feelings, my thoughts. I'm sure there are plenty of other women in my situation who had differ- ent feelings, emotions, thoughts, and anxieties leading up to their sur- geries. We are all unique in how we cope with this difficult decision. After a breast cancer diagnosis, some women will seek out as much information as they can possibly find about their condition through books, the internet, and other sources. Other women, like me, will avoid information altogether in those early stages because it is more than we can process emotionally after the shock of a breast cancer diagnosis.

For previvors, the situation is different because they have not been diagnosed with cancer yet. But many previvors have watched family members struggle with breast, ovarian, and other types of cancers. They may have lost their mothers, sisters, aunts, cousins, or grandmothers to breast cancer already. Men who carry this gene are also at risk for developing breast cancer. Previvors who have tested positive for *BRCA 1* or *2* are typically acutely aware of the risks and this steers their prophylactic mastectomy decisions.

According to estimates of lifetime risk, about 12.0 percent of women (120 out of 1,000) in the general population will develop breast cancer sometime during their lives compared with about 60 percent of women (600 out of 1,000) who have *inherited* a harmful mutation in *BRCA1* or *BRCA2*. In other words, a woman who has inherited a harmful mutation in *BRCA1* or *BRCA2* is about five times more likely to develop breast cancer than a woman who does not have such a mutation. — *National Cancer Institute*[15]

For many previvors, the anxieties associated with ongoing breast surveillance in the form of mammograms, MRIs, and biopsies becomes overwhelming so the decision to have a risk-reducing mastectomy is a welcome relief.

You have to be 110% sure that this is what you want to do. Do it for you and nobody else. I encountered people that thought what I did was not something that they could accept and I got through that by saying to myself that I did this for me and that their opinions did not matter, that I was doing what I needed to do to avoid breast cancer. I received great support from close friends and family and that helped a lot. I also kept a "validation" file where I would put quotes that I found helpful. When I had a down moment I would read it and I would be reminded that what I did was the right thing to do and that I was proud of myself for having the determination to follow through with the surgery and relieve myself of the constant worry of breast cancer. (Sue)

There is a wonderful documentary film called *In the Family* that chronicles the life of a young woman named Joanna Rudnick, the director and subject of the film, as she contemplates risk-reducing surgery after learning that she is *BRCA* positive. This film is powerful in its portrayal of Joanna and other women as they receive their *BRCA* testing results and then sort through the heart-wrenching decisions about prophylactic breast and ovarian surgeries. If you have a family history of breast or ovarian cancer and you are interested in learning more about your risk, see the Resources section for further information about finding a genetic counselor in your area. A genetic counselor will review your family history with you, help you assess your risks, and may recommend further testing when appropriate.

Some of the survivors and previvors I have spoken with have sought mental health counseling to lessen their anxiety about their upcoming mastectomies. If you feel that this would help you, ask your physician to recommend a mental health provider who is well versed in counseling cancer and/or mastectomy patients. To find a provider in your area, contact the American Psychosocial Oncology Society (contact information is listed in the back of this book). There may also be a local cancer support organization that offers group or individual counseling programs that you could attend.

Join a support group!! I didn't think I would need one. But the friendships I developed are great. There really is a need to talk to others who can relate to what you are going through — the tough times as well as laughing at the things that others could not relate to. (Michelle)

Other ideas for reducing anxiety prior to surgery include speaking with other women who have undergone mastectomy and participating in on-line support forums. I love the idea of keeping a "validation file": quotes that you can refer to when the emotional going gets rough. Write in a journal, blog about your experience on-line, do yoga or some other type of exercise to reduce your anxiety, listen to guided imagery. Another veteran shares her strategies for preparing emotionally:

> *Leading up to the surgery, I found the following helpful:*
> *frequent review of why I was doing this (very factual,*
> *specific), meeting with a woman who had had the surgery*
> *with the same surgeon I was using, meeting with another*
> *woman who was scheduled about the same time I was,*
> *having a massage, haircut, and run the day before the*
> *surgery, having meals all lined up for my family. (Kelly)*

And finally, it is important to remember that no one chooses mastectomy lightly, nor should they. There are risks for every type of surgery and your physician should review these risks with you at length. Later on in this book, in the *Voices* section, you will hear from several women who share their own emotional journeys through mastectomy after receiving breast cancer diagnoses and as previvors.

The Big Day Arrives

Now let's discuss the day of the surgery. You have already made the decision to have a mastectomy. And, as much as possible, you have prepared for the surgery both emotionally and physically. The big day arrives and you are a bundle of nerves. If you are having sentinel lymph node mapping done, this may be your first stop. For sentinel lymph node mapping, a series of injections are made in the affected breast using a radioactive tracer and/or a blue dye. The radiologist locates the sentinel lymph node and then marks the skin for the breast surgeon so that he or she can locate it easily for the removal of the sentinel lymph node. I had this procedure done in both breasts prior to my mastectomy and I'm not going to lie — it hurt a lot! At that time there was some controversy over whether or not a local anesthetic should be used for sentinel lymph node mapping because some physicians felt it might compromise the results of the test. Today, nearly three years later, there seems to be a movement to routinely use a topical anesthetic prior to the mapping procedure to help patients avoid unnecessary pain.

Once the sentinel lymph node mapping is completed, you will be ready for the actual mastectomy surgery. I was pretty brave right up until they wheeled me down to the operating room. Then I suddenly became all weepy and overcome with emotion. One of the wonderful nurses held my hand and fetched my husband to wait with me in the staging area outside the operating room. It is hard to describe what goes through your mind when you are waiting to undergo a surgery like this. For me, the emotions that I had kept so tightly hidden over the preceding weeks came rushing forward all at once. But when they finally wheeled me into the operating room and started the anesthesia, I immediately relaxed, felt at ease, and fell asleep. When I woke up a few hours later it felt like only minutes had passed; I was on the "other side" as mastectomy veterans like to call the post-operative phase.

So let's get to the "Now what?" When you wake up after your surgery you will be extremely groggy from the anesthesia and pain medications. You will be hooked up to blood pressure monitors and you will probably have a *PCA — patient controlled analgesic —* pump. It's an IV pump for delivering pain medication that you control by pushing a button on a small hand-held device. This particular machine is pre-programmed by your nurse who has been given specific orders regarding the type of pain medication to be used, the dosage allowed, and the "lock out interval."[16] The lock out interval is the number of doses you can give yourself within a specific time period. In other words, the whole thing is set up so that you can only take the prescribed amount of the pain medicine, so you don't need to worry about over-dosing yourself. I loved that little button! But sometimes narcotic pain medications will cause nausea, which happened to me. Don't hesitate to ask the nurse for something to counteract the nausea. The nurse will run another IV of anti-nausea medication and have you feeling better in minutes. Sometimes the anesthesia and/or caffeine withdrawal will cause headaches. Remember, you probably won't have had your morning cup of coffee or tea on surgery day. If the PCA pump isn't managing your pain adequately, be sure to ask your nurse or physician for additional pain medication so that you are comfortable.

You may have some soreness in your throat after the surgery. This is because during the surgery you were *intubated* — a tube was inserted into your airway to help you breathe during the surgery while under general anesthesia. By the time you wake up from surgery the tube will have been removed and you will be breathing normally again. The soreness in your throat should go away fairly quickly. Drink lots of fluids to soothe your throat and ask your nurse for throat lozenges as needed.

At this stage, you will probably be wearing some type of surgical bra and will have dressings on your incision areas. If you have had a flap surgery you will most likely be attached to a *Doppler ultrasound* machine for the first 24 hours or so. This machine monitors blood flow in your newly transplanted tissue.

On the calf of each leg you will have *intermittent pneumatic compression boots*. These are cloth/Velcro leg wraps that continuously fill with air and then deflate. The compression helps pump the blood back to your heart, thereby preventing blood clots from forming.[17] These wraps can be taken on and off easily. You can also do *ankle pumps* while lying in bed to keep the blood pumping in your legs. With this exercise you just point your toes and then flex your feet back until you feel some stretching in your calf muscles. Try to do this ten times an hour when lying in bed if you don't have your compression wraps on.

You will also be given an *incentive spirometer*. This is a hand-held device to measure inspiratory lung capacity. This helps keep your lungs clear and improves their ability to expand after surgery.[18] Your nurse, physician, or a respiratory therapist will teach you the proper method for using an incentive spirometer. After surgery you should attempt to use the device several times per hour or as instructed by your health care provider. Once you are out of bed and walking the halls on a regular basis, your physician may allow you to discontinue use of the incentive spirometer but be sure to ask before you stop using it. In addition to the incentive spirometer, coughing and deep breathing is encouraged to open up the *alveoli* in your lungs after surgery and reduce the risk of developing post-operative pneumonia.

> ***Hint***: To ease discomfort when coughing, hug a small pillow tightly against your chest.

The New You

When I woke up from surgery I felt a lot of numbness and tightness in my new chest. The feeling was similar to the stiffness you get when you stay in one position for too long. For the first 24 hours or so after my surgery I actually thought I was wearing some type of brace on my torso. I felt like I couldn't really move and I was stiff and sore in my entire trunk.

Years earlier, as an awkward 12-year-old, I had been diagnosed with *scoliosis* or curvature of the spine — yet another gift of my heredity. A special back brace was made for me that went from just under my arms down to my hips. It was made of thick plastic and was cinched in the back — nice and snug — with wide Velcro straps. You can imagine my pre-teen horror at having to wear that thing to school. And pity the poor boy who sat behind me in seventh grade math class and unwittingly allowed his fingertips to drape over the back of my chair, only to have them crushed handily when my brace and I leaned back. When that brace was good and tight, my back was immobile and I would get sore from the lack of movement. And that is pretty much what it felt like when I woke up after my mastectomy. When my plastic surgeon came in the morning after my surgery to remove my bandages and look at his handiwork, it may have been the pain killers talking but I muttered something about being happy to "get this brace off." He must have thought I was crazy, although he politely didn't show it, because that "brace" was my new chest. It was swollen and bruised and it was so firm you could have bounced a quarter off it. My skin and muscles were stretched to accommodate the new implants and this left me with a feeling of extreme tightness in my chest, back, and torso. Another mastectomy veteran who had implant reconstruction describes some of her feelings:

> *I didn't realize how much the implant would feel like a brick lodged in my pec muscle. I wasn't prepared for the extent of the numbness I experienced. (Lynn)*

Another direct-to-implant patient writes:

> *Immediately after surgery I felt like I had a firm/thick pad of some sort adhered to my chest/breast zone. Otherwise I*

felt very good. I would say there was discomfort but not true
pain. (Sue)

Your post-surgical feelings may differ according to the type of reconstruction you have chosen. One veteran who underwent mastectomy
with tissue expander reconstruction describes her feelings:

I felt like my chest weighed 100 lbs! There was so much
pressure that made it hard to breathe, but the narcotics and
pain pump were able to control the pain. I was also
exhausted and slept a ton the first few days! (Amanda)

In addition to the strange physical feelings, there will be some
surprises when you first see your chest after the surgery. One
veteran who underwent mastectomy with DIEP reconstruction says:

I could tell that it was all "me" because I could see some of
the stretch marks that were formerly on my belly were now
part of my new breasts! Yes, my nipples were gone but,
otherwise, I looked down and didn't get a shock because there
were breasts there.

Another veteran who underwent mastectomy with expanders that
were placed immediately writes:

I was greatly surprised when I woke up that I was not
actually flat. I had breasts and while they continued to grow
with each expansion I never felt that I had been disfigured.

No matter what your first glimpse reveals, try not to despair because
it is early yet and your body is responding to the trauma of surgery.
My sister Linda used to say that her newly reconstructed breasts
looked "angry" and that pretty much summed up my experience as
well. There will be lots of bruising, swelling, and discoloration. If
you had nipple sparing surgery, do not be surprised if your nipples
are discolored and peeling for a while. A couple of days after I
returned home from the hospital, I called my plastic surgeon at one
point because I was sure that my nipple — the one that had been
spared — had not actually survived the procedure. He assured me

that it was normal for the nipple to look the way it did, which was dark gray and awful. If you have chosen reconstruction, it isn't until several weeks after surgery, months if you are using expanders, that you will begin to get a sense of what your new breasts will ultimately look like. This great quote from one of the veterans helps keeps things in perspective:

> *Remember that you weren't "perfect" before your surgery,*
> *and won't be after. Everyone is at least a little asymmetrical.*
> *Don't make yourself crazy trying to obtain Hollywood boobs.*
> *Keep your sense of humor. (Sue)*

Truer words have never been spoken. It is important to manage your expectations. If you chose breast reconstruction, there are inevitably going to be dimples, asymmetries, and quirks after the surgery. Remember, none of us chose mastectomy with reconstruction because we wanted to obtain so-called "Hollywood boobs," which is another type of surgery. But that doesn't mean that we don't hope for the best possible outcome. In time, once things have settled down, evened up, and healed a bit, there will be opportunities for your plastic surgeon to give you a nip here or a tuck there. But for now, just concentrate on healing and try to be patient. Remember why you chose a mastectomy in the first place. Lisa describes her feelings after waking up from flap surgery:

> *The moment I woke up from surgery I felt a huge burden*
> *had been lifted from me, and I told whoever was in the room*
> *I'm SO HAPPY! (Lisa)*

Getting Out of Bed

A few hours after your surgery, you may be ready to get out of bed for the first time. Again, depending upon the type of surgery you have chosen, this may or may not be realistic at this early stage. In general, if you have had mastectomy with tissue expander or direct to implant reconstruction, you will be up and about within several hours of your surgery. Most women report taking their first steps between 3 and 12 hours after the surgery. Flap procedures tend to

take much longer to perform. If you have chosen this type of procedure, you will most likely be under anesthesia longer and it may
be a day or so before you are up and out of bed.

It's important to remember: *Always* have a nurse or some other
type of medical professional with you the first few times you try to
get out of bed. When getting out of bed, you should *dangle* your
legs at the side of the bed before you take your first steps. This
means sitting on the side of the bed for a few minutes to let your
blood pressure adjust to the change in body position. Remember,
you have been in bed for a while and your heart doesn't need to
work very hard to pump blood throughout your body when you are
lying down. You have also lost some blood during surgery. If you
move too quickly, before your body has had time to adjust, you
may feel lightheaded or as if you will faint; this is called *orthostatic
hypotension*. So it is important to take it easy and not rush, especially
the first few times you get out of bed.

Some patients report still having a *urinary catheter* at this stage.
A catheter is a tube-like device that is inserted into your urethra so
that your urine drains into a bag. The catheter is usually placed
during surgery. My catheter was removed within a few hours after
surgery. And because of the IV fluids I had been receiving, I
needed to make several trips to the bathroom. The IV pole with
pain pump can be unwieldy and tricky to manage so, again, be sure
to have someone with you to help manage it.

> *Standing and balance were difficult early on in the hours
> post-surgery. Walking was a shuffle with support from
> another person. I was able to use the bathroom myself, but
> needed help getting there for a bit. (Amy)*

A common side effect of catheterization is that, after removal of the
catheter, starting to urinate on your own again can be problematic.
Drinking plenty of fluids can help avoid this problem. If you do
encounter difficulty urinating, sitting on the toilet and concentrating
for a little while with the water running may do the trick but, if not,
be sure to let your nurse or physician know that you are
having difficulties.

It can be very helpful to have someone stay overnight with you
the first night or two in the hospital if possible. Many hospitals

allow this practice, but be sure to ask in advance. My sister MaryBeth stayed with me for both nights in the hospital; it really gave me a sense of calm to have her there with me. If you don't have anyone staying with you, be sure to buzz the nurse on duty whenever you need help.

Once you have made it to the bathroom, keep one hand on the grab bar at all times for safety. This makes clothing management a lot harder than you would expect. Make sure that whatever you are wearing on your bottom half — whether it is just underwear or pajama bottoms — has loose fitting elastic at the waist so you can easily nudge them up and down. This will take some time because, at this stage, your arms and chest will be sore and certain movements will be uncomfortable. My hospital room had an industrial type toilet that I was not able to flush because it took too much strength. After surgery, even this little bit of pressure may be difficult. One mastectomy veteran remarked:

> *It was hard to wipe after using the bathroom! That was a surprise to me! I could not sit up and get out of bed, had to be pushed from behind.*

Using flushable baby wipes instead of toilet paper makes using the toilet a lot easier after surgery.

In the early post-operative hours, you may need a fair amount of help with your basic self-care activities. Just take it slow and ask for help when you need it.

If you have had *sentinel lymph node mapping*, your urine may be blue post-op. This is normal and the color will disappear within a few hours.

Getting to Know Your Post-Op Extras

It is important to remember that everyone's recovery rate and experience will be different depending upon the type of procedure and your age, health status, and activity level prior to surgery. At some point

within the first few post-operative days, unless you have had complications, the IV will be removed and you will be switched to oral pain
medications. Once you are freed from the IV, it is much easier to get
up and move around your room. This is a good time to get to know the
various tubes and drains that are now attached to your body.

You may have a *local anesthetic* that is being delivered by tiny
tubes inserted into your chest area. These are called On-Q
pumps™. The tubes are inserted at the time of the surgery and con-
nected to a fanny pack that contains a *marcaine ball* of anesthetic.
These tubes will stay in place for the next two or three days. Your
doctor will remove the tubes once the anesthetic has run out.
Removal of these tubes is a quick and painless process; I was actually
taught how to remove them myself.

You will usually have two to four *drains* coming out of your
chest, underarm, and/or abdominal areas. The exact location of
the drains will vary according to the type of procedure you have
chosen. If you have had a flap procedure done, you will have
drains at the donor site as well as the reconstruction site. The
purpose of these drains is to collect the excess blood and fluids
after the mastectomy and draw it out of your body. Drain tubes are
typically up to 36 inches long and are attached to a lemon-sized container where the fluid will pool. The containers usually have small
clips so that you can attach them to your bra or another article of
clothing. Do not attach drains bulbs to your pants: If you forget to
unclip the drain bulbs before pulling down your pants, you may
pull out your drains. There is a suture holding the tubing in place
as it exits your chest and underarm area, so it is uncomfortable if
the drains are left dangling or are pulled because they will tug on
your skin. The nurse or physician will teach you how to "strip" or
"milk" the drains so that you can do it yourself once you are discharged. Review the section on drain management later on in this
chapter for more detailed information about handling the drains.

If you have had a direct to implant type of surgery, you may also
have what Linda and I not so fondly refer to as "the strap." The strap
is a long band about two inches wide that wraps behind your back,
under your arms, and across the top of your chest, where it can be
loosened and tightened with Velcro. In other words, it is like a belt
but it is worn just above the bust line. The purpose of the strap is
to help push your implants down so that they eventually settle and

drape like natural breasts. The strap is worn over your bra for the first several weeks after surgery. It is to be worn snug enough so that you can feel it, but not so snug that you can't breathe. The strap ended up being a source of considerable discomfort for both Linda and me. I actually trimmed out the underarms of mine so that it didn't irritate and chafe so much. Sometimes when I was just hanging around the house I would wear it over my clothes because it was just more comfortable that way — definitely a fashion "don't." Occasionally I would remove the strap altogether. The sensory overload of the bra, strap, and whatever healing process was going on sometimes left me feeling like I just couldn't stand it anymore. So I would take off the strap and maybe unhitch the bra for a few minutes just to catch a breather. This happened a lot at night; I would unhinge myself just to take a quick break and inevitably I would wake up several hours later without the strap or bra fastened. I don't recommend this practice necessarily, but I don't think it did any real harm either. You may want to have a conversation with your doctor about what type of realistic wearing schedule is necessary for the strap, if you are given one, as well as for your post-operative bra. Many physicians are now moving away from the strap and recommending a molding bra instead.

Pain and Hydration

During these early post-operative hours and continuing throughout your recovery, it is important to notify your nurse or physician if you are not experiencing adequate pain control. It is normal to feel tightness and discomfort in your chest, shoulders, sides, and even your back after a mastectomy with or without reconstruction. Your health care provider may ask you to rate your pain on a *visual analog pain scale.* This is a standard, self-reporting, pain-rating continuum that ranges from 0 to 10, 0 being no pain, 10 being agonizing pain. Pain is unique because it is subjective. It is not like a blood pressure or temperature reading, which can be measured by instruments. There is no direct measuring device to judge the severity of pain. That means it is up to you to tell your nurse or doctor how "bad" it is. When pain is caused by surgery, pain relief is considered to be a normal part of the treatment. It is a good idea to ask for pain medication before your pain becomes too severe because extreme pain can contribute to shallow breathing and increased fatigue in the post-operative period. It is also harder to get pain under control than it is to head it off in the first place.

It is important to remember to stay hydrated at this stage. One common side effect of narcotic pain medications is constipation. Drinking enough fluids will help counteract constipation. Be sure to ask your nurse for a stool softener like Colace™ if necessary. This will prevent straining and elevation of your blood pressure while using the toilet, particularly important after flap reconstruction. Being proactive about this early on can prevent you from having a lot of discomfort later.

Functioning after Your Surgery

Challenges that many women have reported early in the post-operative period include difficulties reaching for things, getting in and out of bed, getting comfortable in bed, wiping themselves in the bathroom, changing hospital gowns, and pushing the IV pole.

> [*I was*] *unable to do anything myself except push that wonderful bed adjuster button the first day, second day was able to get to bathroom myself, with someone at my side, able to use patient-controlled morphine pump wonderfully! (E.)*

One thing you should know is that almost all hospitals have some type of rehabilitation department. These departments are usually made up of occupational and physical therapists who specialize in helping people get up and around and take care of themselves after illness or surgery in preparation for going home. As an occupational therapist, my job is to make sure that my patients are able to maximize their independence and function safely within the various aspects of their lives after hospitalization. The term "occupation" is used here to describe any purposeful activity that a person might engage in, not just what we traditionally think of as a person's occupation or job. Some of these "occupations" include basic self-care routines like dressing, bathing, and grooming, as well as things like home management and child care. If you are a few days from surgery and you really feel like you could use the expertise of one of these professionals, please do not hesitate to ask your physician to make the referral. During my post-op period, I was not visited by an occupational therapist but I really could have used a *reacher*; this is a long handled device with jaws at the end that helps you pick up objects without bending or straining to reach them. I also could have used some instruction about how to fight my way out that hospital bed. The occupational therapists are also your "go-to" people if you end up needing any kind of *durable medical equipment* when you go home, some helpful equipment includes:

- Shower seat
- Tub or toilet safety grab bars
- Hand-held shower
- Non-skid bath mat
- Reacher

A non-skid bath mat and reacher will probably come in handy for almost everyone. You can buy a non-skid bath mat at any discount department store ahead of time and, in a pinch, a long set of barbecue tongs — as long as they are very lightweight — will do in place of a reacher. If you were an active person going into the surgery and you didn't experience significant complications, chances are that you might not *need* the other devices I have mentioned. That said, it is good to know what to ask for and who to ask if you are feeling at all like you might be at risk of falls in the bathroom/shower area after discharge. Later on in this book, Sara Cohen, OTR/L, CLT-LANA, an occupational therapist specializing in breast cancer rehabilitation at a major cancer center, answers some of the more frequently asked questions regarding rehabilitation needs of women after breast surgery.

Be Your Own Advocate

And this naturally leads me to my next point. I want to say a few words about mastectomy patients and how we may be perceived by hospital staff. There may be a tendency for these professionals to assume that we mastectomy patients know more than we really do. This was my experience but hopefully it will not be yours. Much probably depends upon where you have your surgery. If you are at a major cancer center that sees hundreds of mastectomy patients per year, this may not be your experience. I had my surgery done at a very small local hospital. I was one of two — maybe three — mastectomy patients on the hospital floor at the time. There were lots of other patients on my floor who were not there for mastectomy; many of them were elderly and were there for other medical conditions. I actually felt guilty ringing the nurse call bell because I knew there were other patients on the floor who appeared to need a lot more help and attention than I did. The staff was lovely and helpful, but I got the distinct feeling that they thought I knew more than I really did about what was going on with my surgery and recovery. In general, I think that we mastectomy patients tend to be a fairly well-informed group and we are perceived that way by hospital staff. We are often healthy, vibrant, active women, and we have educated ourselves via books, the internet, and other media sources about breast cancer, mastectomy, prophylactic mastectomy, *BRCA*, and numerous other health-related issues. That was all well and good, but for me — when it came down to the "Now what?" part of this process and getting over the hump of recovery — I needed help. The reason for my long-winded tangent here is to express the following point.

> Ask for information about your specific discharge instructions, follow-up care, do's and don'ts. You will probably be tired and on pain medications at the time of discharge, so you may need to have a friend or family member listen and help you record these instructions. Keep them in a folder marked "hospital instructions."

It is your job to advocate for yourself in getting the information that you need about your recovery. Your physicians may be absolutely the most wonderful people that walk the planet; I know mine were. But they are also human and may not anticipate every last question you will have during the recovery process. And this book will only take you so far because it is nearly impossible to address every single variable that you may be dealing with based on the type of surgery you have chosen and your own physician's rules about the do's and don'ts of recovery. You must be your own advocate and that includes getting the information for discharge from your nurse or physician, recording it carefully or making sure you have been given handouts, and asking follow-up questions when necessary.

> *Don't be afraid to ask questions ... [there is] no such thing as too much information ... even though some may seem overwhelming at the time. My only regret is NOT pushing for more details ahead of time. I would not have changed what I did but it would have made some of it easier to cope with. (Sue)*

And don't be shy about having things explained more than once. It is much better to ask before discharge than to go home and feel that you don't know what you need to be doing or that you are doing something incorrectly. If you are like me, you'll hem and haw about whether or not it is worth contacting your physician because you don't want to "bother" him or her, and so on. Remember this: You are your own best advocate for care and you will need to continue to advocate on your behalf because the process of care and recovery will go on for months on some level. You will probably need to take care of your drains, perform basic wound care, do arm exercises and scar massage, etc., and these things will need to be explained to you along the way. It is important to make time for the necessary discussions between you and your health care providers so that you can take an active role in your recovery.

Preparing for Discharge

This brings us to the topic of hospital discharge. I have mentioned before that your length of stay in the hospital will be based largely on what type of reconstruction you have chosen. If you are having reconstruction with tissue expanders or are going directly to implant, your surgery will typically last for 3–5 hours. Women who undergo these procedures generally tend to have relatively brief hospital stays of 2–3 days, sometimes less. Autologous surgical procedures, reconstruction that uses your own tissue, tend to be longer — sometimes 12 or more hours — so it makes sense that the hospital stay would also be longer. Most women who undergo these types of procedures report being in the hospital for about 4–6 days after surgery.

Before discharge from the hospital, your doctor may apply the post-operative bra you will be wearing for the next several months. Sometimes this is done at one of the early post-op visits. Mine was applied the morning I was discharged. Every physician has his or her own preference for what type of bra is best. Some physicians insist that you wear no bra at all. When a bra is required, typically they are heavy-duty, sports-type bras with good contouring features. Some physicians will tell you *not* to wear anything with an underwire. For the next several days and weeks, unless otherwise instructed by your physician, you will wear this bra 24/7.

Depending upon what type of surgery you had, you may also be given a binder or compression garment to wear. These garments are most often worn on the donor site if you have had a flap procedure. An abdominal binder, for example, may be worn after DIEP or TRAM surgery because these surgeries involve the abdominal area.

You will be given a list of *precautions* or the things you should *not* do. This is an important list. Precautions may involve limits in lifting, arm range of motion, and activity restriction. Here again, your doctor will give you a list of his or her own specific post-surgical rules. Lifting restrictions are prescribed for all types of surgery, though weight limits may differ. Jill describes her precautions:

> *No lifting over 5 lbs for 6 weeks, or raising arms more than 45 degrees from body for first 2 weeks home. No vacuuming. "For how long?" I asked the nurse. "At least a couple of years, right?" "At least," she replied.*

E.'s precautions and recommendations also emphasized movement and lifting restrictions as well as giving her guidance about what her expected activity level should be:

> *No lifting arms above shoulder level, no lifting objects or pulling open doors or using upper body for first week, getting up to move around and walk regularly throughout day encouraged.*

While the drains are in place, some doctors will allow showering while others strictly will not. You will likely be told to keep track of the amount of fluid you are draining from each drain on a daily basis. This will help determine when your drains are ready to be removed. You should be told not to drive while your drains are in or while you are on narcotic pain medications. If your physician does not give you a list of precautions, it is important to ask! The last thing you want to do is open an incision or jeopardize your reconstruction. You can record your precautions and other important information in the chart at the back of this book.

At the time of discharge you will be given instructions about post-operative medications, wound care, and what to watch for in terms of infection and possible complications. If you will be performing wound care yourself, ask your nurse for specific instructions and write them down along with any supplies you will need to purchase. Sometimes the hospital will provide some of the supplies such as gauze bandages. If you have questions about wound care be sure to ask; no question is too simple or obvious at this stage of your recovery. When changing bandages and performing wound care at home, be sure to set up and organize a clean area where you can perform wound care and have access to the supplies you need. Sit down when dressing wounds; this will conserve your energy and if you start to feel faint you will be in a safer position.

One of the most important things to know is what to watch for in terms of red flags in the healing process. Naturally, at this stage, the tissue around your incisions is expected to be pinkish in color and slightly tender. Watch for signs of possible infection, which include:

- Pain
- Redness
- Warm to the touch
- Emitting a foul odor
- Discharge from wound site
- Fever

If you notice any of these conditions after discharge, be sure to notify your physician immediately, as this may indicate complications with your wound healing.

If you have been instructed to use gauze pads or any other type of dressing on your incisions, try to steer clear of using surgical tapes to secure them. Surgical tapes often have adhesives that can cause skin damage to already tender skin. My sister MaryBeth, a seasoned nurse, recommends a product called Surgilast Tubular Elastic Bandage Retainer™. It is a stretchy nylon-elastic blend tubing that comes in all different sizes, including torso size. You can put gauze pads and dressings right under the tubing and they will stay in place. Surgilast may be available in your local pharmacy. If you can't find Surgilast, use a form fitting but not tight tube top as an alternative. Remember to step into the tube top, rather than raising your arms to pull it over your head. The goal here is to avoid the need for surgical tape, leaving your skin free of injuries from the adhesives. If you must use a surgical tape, paper tape is best but be sure to remove it slowly and carefully to avoid causing skin damage.

If your incisions have been covered with *Steri-strips*™ be sure that you do not peel them off. Steri-strips are meant to fall off gradually as the wound heals. If the Steri-strips are peeling and curling at the edges, it is okay to trim them.

Stitches should always be left alone. Most stitches will dissolve on their own as the wound heals. Sometimes a stitch or two will remain and it will feel like a tiny, scratchy bump along your incision. If this happens don't pull on it but be sure to tell your physician so he or she can remove it at a future office visit.

In the hospital you will be given foods that are rich in protein and contain vitamins that promote good wound healing. After discharge you should eat a diet that is high in protein, vitamin C, and vitamin A. Proteins include beans, lean meats, poultry, and fish. Foods that are rich in vitamin A include carrots, leafy greens, butternut squash, dried apricots, and cantaloupe. Foods that are rich in vitamin C include broccoli, cauliflower, leafy greens, oranges, and strawberries.

Make sure to ask your physician when it is appropriate to resume your regular medications. After discharge, call your doctor if you have any questions or concerns about your condition. And be sure to tell your physician if you are not expecting to have any help when you go home. Depending upon insurance coverage you might be eligible to have a home health nurse visit your home to check on your wound healing and drains as needed. Make sure that your physician understands your baseline activity level and your pro-fession. "Resuming normal activities" is different for each patient. A candid discussion early in the process will help remove any con-fusion or miscommunication later on.

Finally, before discharge you should be given information about scheduling your first outpatient appointment with your physician. Try to bring a friend or family member with you to your appoint-ments. Having a second person there with you to take notes or just listen can be helpful. Be sure to write down any questions that you might have ahead of time so that you do not forget them during the appointment.

Drain Management

After discharge from the hospital, your drains will need to be milked 3 or 4 times per day or on the schedule prescribed by your physician. We will all agree that this is not one of the more pleasant jobs you will encounter during your recovery process.

> *My husband ... took care of my drains for me ... those drains coming out of my own body really creeped me out. (E.)*

If you have a family member, friend, or significant other who is willing to jump in and take over here — power to you! Most of us, though, will end up managing the drains ourselves at some point during our recov-ery. I actually preferred to handle them on my own because I was worried about someone else tugging on the tender skin that sur-rounded the area where the tubes came out of my body. If I milked them myself I could stabilize the tube against my body at the top near the suture, so that there was no tugging or pain.

> *I had my husband and mom empty the drains the first few times, but afterwards, I was doing it on my own. It was very easy. (D.)*

Not all hospital discharge instructions are created equal. Some hospitals will provide you with lots information and patient edu-cation materials, while others will not give much. The following are some instructions for managing Jackson-Pratt™ type drains, the type most commonly used after mastectomy.

■ Before you get started, use a permanent marker to label each of your drains 1, 2, 3, etc. This will help you keep track of how much fluid each drain is collecting daily.
■ Gather your supplies ahead of time.
■ Sitting down and having all supplies within arm's reach is recommended prior stripping the drains.

Supplies you will need include:

■ Clean gloves (examination type)
■ Alcohol pads (1-inch square)
■ Plastic container with cc measurements (provided by the hospital)
■ Pencil and drainage chart found at the back of this book

Milking Jackson-Pratt™ type drains[19]:

1. Wash and dry hands thoroughly.
2. Put on clean gloves.
3. Hold the top of drain tube where it comes out of your underarm area with one hand firmly against your torso while using the other hand to draw fluid down the tube into the drainage container. Grip the tube by pinching it between your thumb and index finger. Fold an alcohol pad in half around the tube and use the alcohol pad to help your fingers glide along the tube easily and then wait a few minutes; you are trying to take advantage of the suction the compressed bulb creates. Do not open the bulb stopper when milking the drain.
4. Keeping the spout *closed*, wipe around the outside of the spout with an alcohol pad.
5. Once fluid has moved into the bulb, open the container and pour it into the measuring cup. Do not allow the open spout to come in contact with anything.
6. Squeeze the air out of the container *before* closing the drain. This creates a suction effect that will help with the draining process.
7. Close the spout and then wipe around the outside of the spout with an alcohol pad.

8. Record the amount of drainage in the chart at the back of this book.
9. Repeat this process for all other drains, recording the amount from each.
10. Fluid from drains can be flushed down the toilet.
11. Wash and dry your hands.

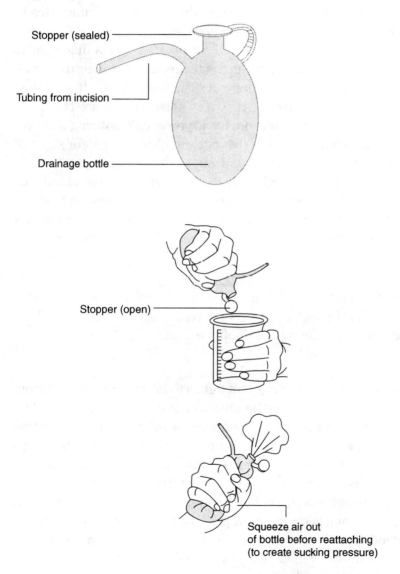

Stopper (sealed)

Tubing from incision

Drainage bottle

Stopper (open)

Squeeze air out
of bottle before reattaching
(to create sucking pressure)

Jackson-Pratt™ Drain.
Courtesy of UCSF Breast Care Center Website.

When you return to your physician for post-operative visits, he or she will use the information you have recorded to determine when the drains are ready to be removed. Fluid will initially be mostly blood or *sanguineous*,[20] indicating that active bleeding is occurring or a *hematoma*[21] is draining. A hematoma is a collection of blood underneath the tissue. The fluid will gradually become more *serosanguineous fluid*,[22] which is pinkish or orangish in color. This type of drainage indicates that healing is occurring and the fluid that accumulates in the mastectomy space is being evacuated. Finally, the fluid will become straw colored; this is called *serous fluid*. This fluid signals that healing is occurring and the drainage process is coming to an end.

Fluid amounts will gradually lessen over time. If drainage amounts increase for a day or two, it is possible you are being too active. Be sure to notify your doctor if you aren't noticing a downward trend in drainage. Watch the incision sites closely for signs of irritation or infection. The wound should be clean and dry; if it becomes red or irritated, call your doctor. Yellow, thick, cloudy, or foul smelling drainage should be reported to your physician immediately as this may indicate infection. If the stitches holding your drains become loose or your drain tube falls out, call your physician.

> It is important that you *never* attempt to clean inside the drain tubing or container as this may cause serious infection. *Do not* attempt to wash out the tubing or bulb.

Here are some really important things to know that many patients are not told: You will *never* be able to completely drain every last speck of fluid or tissue out of the drains or tubes. The drainage will look gross sometimes — that is normal. And do not attempt to clean inside the tubes or drains because, as tempting as this may seem, you open yourself up to serious infection if you do this.

Once drainage has tapered off to a suitable level, usually less than 25–30 cc per drain each day, your physician will remove your drains. It is a good idea to take pain medication prior to drain removal to reduce discomfort. I had two physicians in the room to pull my drains, one on each side of me. They told me to take a deep breath, counted "one, two, three" together, and then pulled. Some people will tell you that drain removal is a breeze but I am not one of them. This actually hurt quite a lot! This not to frighten you but to make the point that there are certain aspects of this process that you will absolutely breeze through, and there are others that you will find surprisingly difficult. The good news was that my pain was short-lived and I felt so thrilled by the prospect of being able to go home and take my first shower in nine days that I quickly forgot about it. Some physicians will ask you to wait a day or two after the drains have been removed before you shower.

One thing to mention here is that I hadn't taken pain medication before the drains were pulled. Actually, I was not a model patient when it came to pain medications during this process. I have always been really hesitant to take medications of any kind because of my slightly irrational fear of allergic reactions. Not that I have ever had an allergic reaction, mind you. Chemotherapy would later cure me of this fear because with chemotherapy you are given steroids, anti-emetics, and what feels like every other medication under the sun just to *prepare* your body for the chemotherapy drugs. At some point, I had to just trust that my medical oncologist knew what he was doing and take all of the medications he prescribed for me. But after my mastectomy, I stopped taking the narcotic pain medications about 12 hours after surgery and moved right to the heavy duty Tylenol™. In retrospect, this was probably not one of my better decisions.

As I mentioned earlier, I was lucky that my pain level with the mastectomy was never very high. For me it was more discomfort based on stiffness, tightness, and being somewhat immobile. But I *did* have discomfort and I really did not sleep well for several nights after the surgery. Although this is normal to some degree, I think that if I had been a little more generous with my pain medications I could have avoided having so much discomfort and so many sleepless nights that first week or so. Getting a good night's sleep might have helped lift my spirits during that time as well. Listen to this advice from one of the mastectomy veterans:

[A mastectomy] hurts. Take pain meds as often as needed. You don't get a medal or any extra credit for needless suffering. It's not actually as easy to get addicted as most people fear, and your doctor will tell you if that's a concern. (Jill)

Bed Mobility and Sleeping

This brings us to bed mobility and sleeping. Occupational and physical therapists love to talk about bed mobility with their patients. And if you think about it, moving in bed is an important skill to learn after any type of surgery. Getting in and out of bed can be *really* difficult during the first few days after surgery. Your shoulders, chest, and abdominal muscles may be sore. If you have had a flap procedure, the donor site will be sore as well. One thing you should know is that hospital beds are not made for getting in and out of easily. If you raise the head of the bed to help you get a head start on sitting up, make sure to lower the foot of the bed. If you don't do this you create a large crevice for your rear-end that is nearly impossible to get out of. That said, silky pajama bottoms can be helpful in easing bed mobility because they slide along the sheets easily.

> *Get help when needed, sleep on your back (the only position you can), make sure drains are secure and (for implant reconstruction) move using your stomach muscles, as chest/shoulder muscles are of no help for a while.*

Another veteran shares her experience:

> *I learned to drop my feet off the side of the bed and brace them against the side of the bed to move me to an upright position. I had my oopherectomy three weeks after prophylactic bilateral mastectomy, so I was advised not to use my abdominals for a while, which made changing positions a creative dilemma. (E.)*

Here are a few things to remember about bed mobility:

- If you have had a *left* breast mastectomy, it is best to exit from the right side of the bed.
- If the surgery was on your *right* breast, exit from the left side of the bed.
- If your surgery was *bilateral* or on both sides, exit from either side of the bed using the same technique given below.

The best option for getting out of bed is as follows:

1. To begin, bend the knee that is farthest away from the side of the bed you plan to exit. Use this leg to push off and gently roll to your opposite side. Make sure you are hugging a pillow here so that you aren't tempted to overuse your affected arm or arms and to help with pain associated with the movement. It is possible to bear most of the weight on your hip as you roll, making it more like a segmental lower body roll. This leaves mostly your hip and the back of your shoulder to bear the weight of your body against the mattress.

2. Next, bend both knees and swing your legs over the side of the bed. This will help counterbalance your upper body weight, making it easier to sit up. Use your calves and thighs against the edge and side of the bed to sit up. This might require some practice ahead of time. If you have had flap surgery like a DIEP or TRAM that left you with an abdominal incision, you may have limitations in your abdomen right after surgery so your leg strength is going to be really important. If you have had a single mastectomy, you can obviously use your unaffected arm to help you sit up.

Try to practice using this method before your surgery so you get a feel for how to do it. Remember that there is no shame in needing help with bed mobility in the days immediately following surgery.

Remember: You should not be strenuously pushing or pulling with your arms when sitting up as this may jeopardize your incisions or reconstruction.

During the first days and weeks post-surgery, sleeping can also be a challenge. Some of us find it difficult to sleep on our backs but this is the best option for post-mastectomy patients. You will probably need a lot of pillows or a foam wedge to prop yourself in a semi-upright position for comfort. Some people choose to sleep in a recliner after surgery; if you don't own one, it is possible to rent a recliner from a medical supply company.

Sleeping in a recliner was the only way for me, I lived in mine for at least 4 weeks in fact. Later, I found an extra long "body pillow" (that) helped to support me in a comfortable angle. (Jill)

Sleeping flat on my back after surgery was simply not an option because of the discomfort I felt in my chest and torso. I didn't have a recliner but my bed was pushed into a corner so I was able to prop myself up with pillows and wedge myself in the corner for back support. One of those donut-shaped neck travel pillows would have really come in handy. Also a "husband" pillow, a back pillow with small arms rests, would have been nice. Many women swear by the Leachco Back-N-Belly Pillow™ pictured here and listed in the resources section at the back of the book.

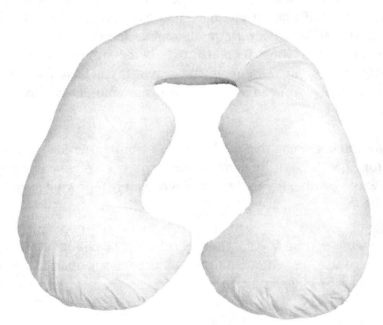

Leachco™ Back-N-Belly Pillow.
Photo courtesy of Leachco.

Whatever you choose, you should also keep your arms elevated on pillows to reduce the risk of lymphedema. As mentioned, lymphedema is swelling that can occur in your arms after lymph node removal associated with mastectomy. I will go into more depth about lymphedema later on in this book. One of my physicians has manufactured her own line of mastectomy products including the Axilla Pilla™, designed for use after mastectomy to reduce soreness in the underarm area, also called the axilla.

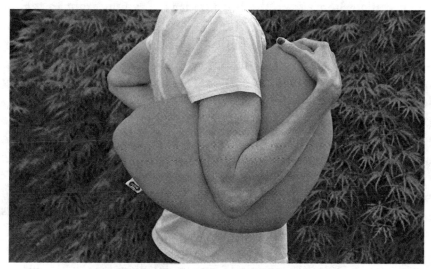

Axilla Pilla™. Courtesy of Best Friends for Life Co.

One mastectomy veteran recommends putting an extra quilt on the bed to give the mattress added cushioning and sleeping in a twin bed so that it is easier to get in and out. Pillows under your knees will help prevent you from sliding down in the bed when you are lying down.

During recovery I slept in bed, semi-reclining on a stack of pillows. It took 2–3 nights to work out how to get the pillows just right. I wish I'd experimented before the surgery, as dealing with the pillows afterwards was a source of considerable frustration. Could have experimented beforehand when I had better mobility to adjust things. (Liz)

Experimenting with the pillows ahead of time is good advice. Before your surgery, be sure to set up your sleeping area with pillows and practice getting in and out of the bed using some of the bed mobility techniques listed earlier.

Your Activity Level after Discharge

Once you get home from the hospital it is very important to take it easy. This doesn't mean that you should be lying in bed all day but too much activity isn't a good idea either. In the beginning, for me, walking from one end of my living room to the other was cause for me to sit down and take a breather. That was incredibly frustrating for me. After about four or five days of being home, and gradually pushing myself a bit further each day, we went to the track at the local elementary school. I walked halfway down the length of one side of the track before I had to pull up to sit on a bench. This was one of the most depressing moments of my recovery. I just wasn't bouncing back fast enough. My surgeon had explained to me that I had lost a lot of blood and I guess that, combined with all of the stress leading up to the surgery, had really worn me down. I was also at my thinnest point in my adult life, mostly due to having no desire to eat after the shock of my initial diagnosis. This weight loss added to my overall physical weakness and low endurance. Gradually, over a period of a few weeks, I was able to walk several laps around the track before fatiguing. You need to ask your doctor how much activity you should be expected to do those first couple of weeks. My advice is to try to take a short walk every day. Before long you will see that you are able to make it farther and farther, in small increments, before you fatigue. Be sure to bring someone with you when you go out for a walk so that, in the unlikely event you run into trouble and aren't feeling well, you are not out there by yourself. I was not in stellar shape cardio-wise before I had the surgery but neither did I get out of breath easily just from walking, so it really concerned me when my endurance was so low that I couldn't even walk the length of a track without sitting down. Many women who I have spoken with exercised more intensely in the days and weeks leading up to their surgeries. These women often described fairly easy recoveries and many felt that this could be attributed to their fitness level going into the surgery. One physician friend, an avid marathoner, was out running two weeks after her surgery. She wore two bras to support her healing chest. That doesn't mean that you should go out and run two weeks after surgery, but it does illustrate that there is a wide range in what is considered a "typical" rate of recovery.

But let's not get ahead of ourselves here. The first few days after discharge you will still feel fatigued, lack energy, and may become short of breath easily. As one mastectomy veteran remarked:

> *I found I could only do one thing a day for a while. Going to the grocery was an exhausting process. (Debbie)*

Energy Conservation

To prevent yourself from getting too worn out during daily activities, you need to practice *energy conservation* techniques, common-sense principles for reducing the amount of energy the body expends on a daily basis doing things like basic self-care, work, and home management tasks. These techniques can be incorporated into your daily life during the first days and weeks after your surgery; they include[23]:

- Pace yourself, do not rush.
- Plan ahead, organize, and schedule your day ahead of time.
- Gather all the supplies you need for each task before you start: dressing, bathing, cooking, etc.
- Use a reacher for hard-to-reach objects but do not attempt to lift heavy objects.
- Take frequent rest breaks; this will help save energy for other activities you enjoy.
- Alternate light and heavy tasks throughout the day and week.
- Sit while working whenever possible.
- Don't overuse your arms. Excessive arm movements, in addition to possibly breaking your precautions, will cause you to fatigue more quickly.

If you start to feel light-headed or clammy with a rapid heartbeat, this is a sign of low blood pressure or low blood sugar. Make sure you have someone in the house in case you feel faint.

In general, you are going to want to pare down your self-care routine after surgery. I like this advice from one of the veterans who underwent mastectomy with expanders:

Simplify your self-care routine as much as possible — just like after having a baby, it's a good day if you can brush your teeth and hair. (E.)

Bathing

Check with your physician about bathing restrictions during the post-operative period. If you are not permitted to shower while the drains are in place, you may consider using dry shampoo, having a family member or friend wash your hair for you in the sink, or making an appointment for a hair wash and blow dry at a local salon.

Even if you're bathing alone, have someone on standby, it is surprisingly hard to get in and out when you're not supposed to bear weight on your arms. Having your hair washed and clean makes you feel really good — if you can't do it, go to a salon or have a friend/spouse do it. It's a mood lifter. (Kelly)

My drains were in for nine days during an April heat wave so my husband washed my hair in the kitchen sink. It was great for my psyche. One mastectomy veteran's husband helped her wrap her chest in plastic wrap to cover all of the incisions and drains so that she could shower: "Not elegant but effective," she said. Desperate times will occasionally call for desperate measures. Another veteran wrote:

I had my husband wash my hair the first week I was home, and that did wonders for me. [I] purchased a shower seat to sit on so he could wash me and my hair without getting my incisions wet. (E.)

A sponge bath while sitting at the sink or just using baby wipes may be the best option for cleansing your body without breaking the rules. Lotions, powders, and deodorants should not be used near incisions until they are fully healed.

Many women recommend that you have your underarms waxed or lasered before surgery to prevent hair from bothering you, to prevent odor, and to lessen the risk of infection from shaving. This is especially good advice if you will be recovering during warm weather.

Once you are allowed to bathe, a hand-held shower may be helpful. Leave the shower head hanging down between uses so that you don't have to lift your arms overhead to reach it. If the drains are still in, use a lanyard or shoelace tied around your neck to hook the drains to. Be sure to have a non-skid mat in place and don't try to shower without having someone on standby for safety.

Before getting in the shower for your first post-mastectomy shower, make sure everything you need is available at a low level. I could not reach up and all my favorite soaps/ shampoos were over my head and inaccessible. (Sue)

Here are some energy conservation tips for bathing:

- Gather all items for dressing and bathing in one area before you begin.
- Sit while bathing if possible.
- Use a hand-held shower and/or shower stool if necessary.
- Do not use water that is too hot; this increases fatigue and can cause hypotension/fainting.
- After bathing, sit while drying yourself.

Finally, for safety's sake, never use towel racks or built-in soap dishes to support your weight like you would tub or toilet grab bars. Towel racks and soap dishes are not meant to support significant amounts of weight and likely will pull out of the wall. There are specific types of tub grab bars that can be clamped on the side of the tub and adjusted as necessary. This type of grab bar is good because it can easily be clamped on and then removed when you no longer need it. Review the equipment list in the Functioning After Surgery area for more information.

Dressing

Dressing yourself can also present challenges after surgery. After a mastectomy it is important to choose clothing that is loose fitting. Tops should be button front or zipper front, with extra room to accommodate dressings and drains. Listen to this advice from one of the mastectomy veterans:

> *Front button shirts or really loose ones with wide neck*
> *openings and stretchy material, and elastic pants — no*
> *buttons or zippers to mess with — yoga pants worked great*
> *for me. Shoes that don't need to be tied or buckled, that you*
> *can just slip your feet into. A fanny pack to carry essentials*
> *in, as wearing a shoulder strap can be uncomfortable.*

Some people choose to wear all of the drain containers in a waist pack, rather than clipping them inside their clothing. I did this for a while and it worked pretty well. Once the On-Q™ local anesthetic had run out and been removed, I then used the fanny pack it had been in to hold all of my drains. There are also special mastectomy camisoles with built in pouches for the drains. I never tried one of these but certainly would have had I known about them.

> *Check with [your] insurance [company] if mastectomy bras*
> *or camisoles are covered. I got 2 bras and 2 camisoles*
> *paid for by insurance. Two of them had drain holders which*
> *were SO convenient. (Amy)*

Each person has her own preference for what works best. What works great for one person might be less effective for another:

> *I bought a mastectomy camisole, but found it pretty useless.*
> *Pinning the drains to my clothing, or putting them in*
> *my hoodie or sweats pockets worked fine… I wore*
> *camisoles/tanks that I could slip on over my feet, and then*
> *wore a zip up hoodie. (Kelly)*

Your physician may ask you to buy your post-operative bra before your surgery. Each physician has his or her own preference for what bra is best depending upon what type of surgery you choose. If you are unsure about fit, try to buy more than one size ahead of time and then ask your physician to help you choose which one provides the best fit and contour. Leave tags on and save receipts so that you can return the unused bra later on.

Except for the two bras I bought ahead of time and paid for out of pocket, I really didn't invest in anything special for my surgery. I have since learned that Medicare and most private insurance companies will cover a portion of the bras and prosthetics you may need following your surgery. Medicare covers these supplies at the rate of 80 percent. Check with your private insurance company to see what their coverage rate is for these items; it should be comparable. Medicare covers the following:

- Two post-operative camisoles within the first 90 days after surgery
- Seven mastectomy bras every six months

There are companies that specialize in selling mastectomy supplies such as bras, breast forms, and nipples. You may need a physician's prescription in order for these items to be covered by insurance. In some cases, the bra company will help you determine your eligibility and then will do all the Medicare or insurance paperwork for you. There is more information about prosthetics in the next chapter.

When putting on a bra, it is easiest if you first clip it around your waist with the fastener in the front. Then rotate the fastener to the back; gently slide your affected arm into the strap first before pulling the bra into position. Remember to always dress your affected arm first because it has less range of motion right now. If you had bilateral surgery, just put both arms in the straps and gently pull the bra into position. If you can find a suitable bra that fastens in the front, that's even better.

On your bottom half you'll need pants with an elastic waist so that they are easy to pull up and down, "yoga"-type pants are perfect. Button front and zipper pants, like jeans, can be challenging and painful to negotiate right after surgery so they are not recommended at this stage. This may be particularly true if you have had tissue expander or implant surgery, which disrupts the pectoralis muscles and makes some of the movements at midline, like zippering and buttoning pants, uncomfortable. In terms of footwear, slip-on shoes are easiest to manage because bending over to tie shoelaces can be challenging.

> Wear loose fitting clothing that doesn't take a lot of energy to put on. This will also help with drain management.

When getting dressed, here are a few basics to keep in mind:

- Gather all of the clothing you will need and place it within arm's reach.
- Sit while dressing for safety and energy conservation purposes.
- Always dress the affected arm first because it has less range of motion or ability to move freely.
- Dressing your upper body uses more energy, so do this first.[24]
- Put underwear and pants on together to avoid bending, standing, and pulling up more than once.
- When dressing your lower body — underwear, pants, socks — bring each foot up to the opposite knee in order to prevent excessive forward bending.

Remember, you can ask the hospital's occupational therapist to provide a *reacher*. This can be helpful with dressing activities including putting on pants. If lower body dressing is really a struggle for you after your surgery, also ask your occupational therapist about a *sock aid*, *dressing stick*, and/or *long handled shoehorn*. These items can be very helpful if reaching your feet is a challenge after surgery.

Home Management

Try to get your household ready ahead of time. In the kitchen, put frequently used items at waist level and well within reach. Instead of lifting heavier items, slide them along the counter.

Put necessities on the counter or below the counter —
nothing in cabinets above the counter that you have to reach
up to. Buy juice/milk in sizes no larger than pint or half
gallon, as it may be too heavy to lift. Don't expect to be able to
use a can opener, chop veggies, push a vacuum cleaner, push
a heavy shopping cart. (E.)

You probably won't be feeling up to doing regular chores after
discharge — nor should you — so your house might not be too
clean for a while. Try to accept this fact, especially if you have
kids. This is another time when managing expectations becomes
important. I was lucky to have my surgery during the spring when
my husband's work schedule is much less busy than at other times
of the year. He was able to be home a lot and he could drive me to
my medical appointments. He did his best to keep up with the housework but because we have fundamentally different ideas of the
concept of "clean" — as many husbands and wives do — I had to
bite my tongue from time to time. In the end, I had to put housework
in the category of things that I was just going to have to let go for a
while. This was not an easy thing to do, believe me. Just to preserve
my sanity a little bit, when I was feeling up to it, I would walk around
the house with my reacher and pick up lightweight items like toys
and clothes, that had been left on the floor. As much as possible
you should attempt to delegate to your partner and other family
members. Try to make chore charts and offer rewards or extra allow-
ance to children as needed. And remember that this is a temporary
condition for you. It may take several weeks before you are up to
speed but you will get there.

Because getting out to shop for groceries may be difficult, look
into home delivery or have someone shop for you. I did some
research on the grocery stores in my local area and found that
almost all of them offer some type of on-line ordering service and
some of them deliver free of charge. If you must go to the store, try
to bring a friend with you, and go during off-hours — there will be
fewer people and your chances of getting bumped into are less.
Something to avoid early in your recovery period are crowded
areas where you run the risk of getting bumped or jostled. Have a
friend or a willing stock person push the grocery cart for you. Put
only a few items in each grocery bag to keep the weight down and

ask for help getting heavier items in and out of the cart and in and out of your car. Make sure to ask for help pushing the cart to your car, opening the trunk, and loading the car.

Instead of cooking, make and freeze meals before your surgery or stock up on frozen or canned foods that will be easy to cook. If you have support from family and friends, you might want to set up a calendar and ask people to sign up to provide meals for you and your family the first week or two after discharge.

> *If you live alone, buy paper plates and plastic utensils so you don't have to do dishes ... get groceries delivered; hire someone to clean the cat box or take the dogs for a walk if you can't. (Brenda)*

When doing laundry, be sure not to carry heavy laundry baskets. When loading the washer or dryer, place items in one or two at a time so as not to break your lifting restrictions. Buy individual detergent packets or scoopable powder ahead of time; a big plastic jug of detergent will be too heavy for you to handle after surgery.

> *Accept HELP! So many women think they have to be superwoman ... I couldn't have done it without the help of friends to do laundry, shop, etc. The thing is that they WANT to help — it makes them feel better and when you don't accept the help, you are denying them that AND you are threatening your own recovery. (Geri)*

Folding laundry may be very manageable but be sure not to break movement restrictions, lift heavy items, or wear yourself out too much. Again, if your endurance is an issue, be sure to pace yourself and limit arm movements to avoid excessive fatigue.

Caring for Children

If you have children, the issues are really twofold. First, how do you help them cope emotionally with your surgery? And second, how do you care for them after your surgery?

First, the emotional part; try to prepare them ahead of time for what to expect and how they can help you during your recovery.

You don't need to go into a lot of detail here; just provide them with the basics of what they need to know explained in a way that they can understand and that isn't too scary for them. Respond to questions succinctly but without giving a lot of extra unnecessary information. In general, I like this advice from Nancy, one of the mastectomy veterans, about how to help your children cope with mastectomy:

> *Keep their lives as normal as possible. Don't involve them in discussions/decisions about treatment, tell them what they can understand at their developmental level in a matter of fact way so they won't become scared.*

Enlist children to help you during your recovery. Some children will relish the idea of being able to help take care of Mommy and you might find them to be surprisingly gentle. When my sister Linda was napping one day during her recovery at my house, my three-year-old Claire ever-so-gently spread her "blanky" — her most prized possession — over Linda to keep her warm and comfortable. After my surgery, we told Claire that, like Auntie, I had "boo boos" so I wasn't going to be able to lift her up and I would have to take it easy for a while. She understood this and was very patient and careful with me. Teach kids ahead of time about gentle hugs. We enjoyed lots of hugs but I always kept a small pillow between us for my protection.

To my older daughter, Phoebe, who was eight years old at the time of my surgery, we explained that I was going to be getting the same surgery as Auntie Linda. Because she had watched Linda's recovery — and seen her up and about, fully dressed, and functioning somewhat normally within a couple of days — she understood that this was not a "big, scary operation" that was going to leave Mommy out of commission for weeks or months on end. We explained it to her in a very matter-of-fact way and she accepted it, as such, without difficulty. As the years have progressed and her ability to understand and process information has increased, I have offered information in more detail whenever she inquires.

I am not an expert in the area of mental health or counseling but my very wise and wonderful mother-in-law Nancy Baker, who is a clinical social worker with years of experience counseling children and families, once told me that "Our children are barometers for how we, as adults, are doing emotionally." I believe this to be true now that I have seen it played out time and time again in my own family. When I'm stressed out my kids are unhappy, they can be difficult to manage, and I see a lot more negative behaviors. When I'm happy, calm, and stress free, my kids tend to be much more positive, happy, and easy-going themselves. So if you are stressed out and struggling to deal with a mastectomy and/or a cancer diagnosis, then chances are that your kids are probably struggling, too. They may not be showing it in the same way an adult would, but sometimes behaviors will appear that may be a result of some internal stress they are feeling. And just like you may need to seek counseling or find relaxation techniques, they may also have these needs. Your best bet is to give kids an opportunity to talk about their concerns, read books that relate to what they may be going through, and if need be, follow up with a mental health professional who can counsel them appropriately.

When I was going through my mastectomy and then chemotherapy, I felt very thankful when friends or family members would offer to take my kids for a day or an afternoon. It wasn't so much that I wanted to get the kids out of my hair, it was because I wanted them to have a good time and get away from their reality for a while. My sister MaryBeth and my Mom were wonderful at keeping the kids occupied and entertained during their visits. But there were also times when it was just us and I wasn't feeling up to caring for them or spending time with them; then they would just mope around the house or watch television and that made me so sad. If friends and family want to help, ask them to take your kids for an hour or two — to the library, the local playground, or just outside to play in the backyard. It will help you feel better and will give your kids a nice break.

Now to address the actual physical demands of taking care of a child after surgery; if you have small children, you will almost certainly need to enlist the help of family, friends, and reliable babysitters after your mastectomy. My sister Linda's daughter was less than a year old when Linda had her surgery. Because Linda had traveled from Hawaii to New York for her mastectomy, she ended up being separated from the baby for nearly two weeks. As tough as it was on both of them, Linda feels that it helped her get a jump-start on healing. Once she returned home to Hawaii, she set up a futon on the floor so that they could snuggle easily and without a need for lifting.

You will need help. There is no way around this if your children are small. Mine are 4 years old and 2 years old. Before my surgery, we practiced how we could snuggle without touching my chest. We do leg hugs and hand hugs instead of full hugs.

Another veteran with small children shares her experience here:

Send her to daycare! I stayed at my brother's house for the first week, since we live 2 hours from the hospital. My daughter stayed with my husband. I missed her terribly, as that was the longest we've ever been apart, but I think it was psychologically better for both of us. She didn't see the worst of it. She did ask me if the drains were juice boxes! She's almost three, so she can get herself onto the toilet and into bed. I really don't know how I would have done it if she were younger.

For babies, diapering can be done on a towel or changing table cushion set up on the floor so that you don't have to do any lifting. If you have a toddler who is on the move, changing the diaper while he or she is standing can also work.

Try to rethink how you do things prior to surgery — [set up a] diapering station on the floor, a feeding chair with seatbelt on a splat mat, ... transition to showering for old enough children. Get children accustomed to snuggling with you while you have a pillow between your chest and them. Promote your children's independence in daily activities with great fanfare! (Lynn)

For older kids, one of the veterans recommends getting your kids involved in your healing process and writes:

My boys were seven at the time. Involving them in helping seemed to take the fear out of it for them. They would bring

me drinks, open or close the recliner for me and rub my feet.
I was very blessed ...

For your children's sports and activities, set up a ride schedule ahead of time. Enlist friends, family, and other parents to carpool and give rides as needed.

Let someone else do it for at least 2 weeks!!! Make sure
someone is scheduled to drive them to soccer or whatever.
I was also careful to wear makeup and dress nice after a
couple days so they would see their Mommy looking rela-
tively healthy and good, even if I was sitting on the couch.
Teach everyone about "hospital hugs" where you hug but
don't press at the chest, good advice for any kid to know how
to hug without hurting. (Frances)

Managing expectations is also important when it comes to your children's activities. These days many children are involved in numerous after-school clubs and activities. As much as you want to and should try to keep your children's routines as normal as possible during this time, if you are unable to drive them here, there, and everywhere and carpooling isn't an option, they may have to take a break from activities for a couple of weeks. This can be a really tough pill to swallow for you and your kids because Moms tend to try to be superwomen and our kids tend to think we *are* superwomen. In the year following my diagnosis, when I was returning to work after six months off for my surgery and chemotherapy, I made a conscious decision to take it easy. For me, this meant not running my children to dance class, horseback riding lessons, and so on several days a week after work. And as much as possible I did my best to remain guilt-free about this decision. This was my gift to myself and the truth is that my kids really didn't seem to care; we have never returned to our pre-cancer involvement level when it comes to the kids' activities. The moral of my story: Taking a couple of weeks off from toting your kids around to one activity after another is not going to be the worst thing that ever happened to them. And, who knows, you may end up finding some hobbies or activities that you enjoy doing at home together.

Driving

Driving is generally not permitted until your drains have been removed. This is because of the risk of accidents and because any quick jerk of the steering wheel might cause you to dislodge a drain tube or suture, setting your recovery back needlessly. It is also important that you have stopped using the narcotic pain medications before you begin driving again. Once your physician clears you to drive, a car that has automatic transmission is certainly a lot easier to handle than a manual transmission that requires use of a stick shift. I remember that my sister Linda had a hard time releasing the emergency brake on my car — she couldn't do it without breaking her precautions.

After surgery you will probably want to have some type of cushioned shoulder strap cover for your seat belt. If you are handy, you can sew one yourself with a soft fabric like faux lamb's wool or fleece. Another option is to use a small pillow, like the Axilla Pilla™, between you and the shoulder strap to prevent discomfort.

Your Emotions after Surgery

Emotionally, the first week or so after surgery was probably the toughest for me. As I have said, I didn't have the energy I would have expected and my emotions seemed to be all over the place.

Obviously, undergoing a mastectomy is a major psychological stressor. And one can't help but also question whether or not the physiological changes associated with mastectomy — perhaps including hormonal fluctuations — may impact on our feelings of emotional well-being in those early post-operative days and weeks. Many women report having hot flashes after mastectomy; these can contribute to feelings of irritability and discomfort.

This can be a tough period to endure; you may have feelings of loss, grief, and/or isolation. Be sure to speak with your physician about how you are feeling emotionally at your post-operative visits.

About two weeks after the surgery, I found that I was feeling pretty good and getting back to my normal self again both emotionally and physically. The removal of the drains really is a turning point in recovery because it often marks your ability to begin to bathe, dress normally, drive a car, and otherwise feel human again.

Once you have reached this point you will likely feel that you have reached a tremendous milestone in your recovery. Congratulations! However, if complications or pain issues persist, this process may be delayed, which can be tremendously frustrating.

In the next chapter I will address many of the mastectomy aftercare issues including range of motion exercises, being fitted for a breast prosthesis, performing scar massage, what to expect in terms of sensation, lymphedema prevention, nipple reconstruction, going back to work, and more. I will also address some of the "what ifs" related to complications and pain.

3

After-Care, Recovery, and Complications

Sensation

Sensation is subjective and will be different for every person after a mastectomy with or without reconstruction. I have already talked about what the initial physical feelings and sensations were like after my mastectomy with direct to implant reconstruction tightness, discomfort, and muscle stiffness in my chest, trunk, and back, as well as some *phantom sensation*. Phantom sensation is well documented in individuals who have lost all or part of a limb due to amputation. These sensations can include feelings of pain or itching in the extremity, even though the extremity is no longer there. It turns out that mastectomy patients can experience phantom sensation as well. My phantom sensation consisted of itching that lasted on and off for a few months after my surgery. It was mostly aggravating–I couldn't localize the itch and no amount of scratching would give me relief because I couldn't feel the scratching!

As the weeks and months passed after my mastectomy, I came to realize that the skin sensation in my chest was all but gone and this might be a more or less permanent situation. Return of sensation after mastectomy with and without reconstruction is something that varies greatly according to procedure. Many women report no return of sensation; others experience fairly good return of sensation. Much depends upon the extent of nerve damage that you sustain in the process of the mastectomy.

Every now and again, when I visit my surgical oncologist for my follow-up visits, he pulls out a pin and starts poking me to see what type of sensation I have in my breasts. Around the periphery and in between my breasts my sensation is essentially normal but anything interior, toward the nipple area or on the breast mound proper, has no feeling. Certain areas of my underarms, rib cage area, and a small area of my back behind my left armpit also have limited or no sensation. I really don't mind this lack of sensation and I choose to compartmentalize this particular inconvenience as being a sign of a job "well done" by my surgeon. This certainly does not mean that if you have a return of sensation, your surgeon was less than thorough in his technique. That is not the case at all. Sensory nerves are cut during the procedure as a necessary part of removing all the breast tissue. No critical motor or sensory nerves are cut during a mastectomy. The sensory impact of the surgery varies according to variability of regrowth of nerves and of adjacent intact nerves cross covering the area. As nerves regenerate or grow back, they will do so at a very slow rate — approximately one millimeter per day. My sister Linda who, you will remember, had essentially the same surgery as I did although hers was prophylactic, experienced a gradual but incomplete return of sensation over the past three years. So you see, every person's experience is different. And similarly, every woman will have a different emotional response to losing or having diminished sensation. Some women find it deeply upsetting to lose this sensation while others find it of little consequence.

For many couples, breast stimulation is an important part of lovemaking and provides a source of great sexual pleasure. Nipple stimulation is known to cause the release of the oxytocin hormone in the brain that plays a role in sexual arousal and — though the exact mechanism is not fully understood — is thought to be related to orgasm. After mastectomy these nerve pathways are disrupted and breast sensitivity is decreased or eliminated permanently. The degree of loss of sensitivity is dependent upon the type of surgery as well as some individual differences, but after a major surgical procedure such as this, the changes are usually substantial and the return of erotic sensation in that area is unlikely.

Other factors in post-mastectomy sexuality go far beyond the anatomy and physiology of the reconstructed/non-reconstructed breast area. These factors include a woman's perception of her own cosmetic outcome, partner reaction, health, psychological status, whether or not there is residual pain, on-going radiation or chemotherapy, or use of medications that decrease estrogen levels.

Body image may play one of the most important roles in post-mastectomy sexuality. How we feel about this "new self" can influence our intimate lives immensely.

As healing progresses, each individual is bound to experience the return of sensation differently. Kim reports how she felt 12 days after her mastectomy with tissue expanders before her fills began:

> *Lots of tingling and tightness in the chest. Sore and sensitive in the armpit area. In the beginning it was like a heavy weight on my chest, now at 12 days post-op the weight has eased up but the back pain has been challenging ... aside from certain areas at the top and bottom of my breasts, most of all the skin is numb.*

Amy reports on her sensation three months after her initial surgery with tissue expanders placed and eventual exchange to implants:

> *Initial surgery, almost 13 weeks ago. Exchange 5 days ago. No sensation on my breasts. Above my breast and below my collar bone, I have a tingly, "asleep-like" feeling in my skin. I am not expecting feeling although it would be a lovely surprise.*

And here, Sue reports on her sensation eighteen months after her mastectomy with direct to implant reconstruction:

> *I have no feeling in my breasts but [in] all other areas I do have feeling, upper chest, below breasts. I have no problem with the sensation that I have and I'm sure that no more will return.*

Nearly eight years after DIEP flap surgery, Tara describes sensation at both her donor site and her reconstruction site:

> *The area where the flap was taken is numb.... Outside of the scar and the new belly button the donor site has no*

*long-lasting effects.... When feeling started to return to my
breast it was uncomfortable. I started getting itchy and then
I would start feeling something like a jolt of electricity
almost like when a body part falls asleep and then the feeling
starts to return. I know that I have more feeling in my
breasts because I have found myself pulling away from a hot
towel rack without realizing my breast was almost touching. I felt the heat and I know that it was something that I
had not felt for some time after surgery.*

About six months after my mastectomy, I went back into surgery
to have the nipple reconstruction done on my right breast. At no point
during my recovery from the nipple reconstruction, or the areola
tattoo that followed a few months later, did I experience any pain
or other sensation to the reconstructed nipple area. It was numb,
completely numb. So with that in mind, when I went back for a revision of my areola tattoo last year, I declined the local anesthetic that
is routinely given to mask the pain of the tattooing process. To my
shock and delight, I felt that tattoo being put on and it actually
kind of hurt! I could feel both pain and the vibration of the instrument
as the tattoo was applied. So within the course of one year, and two
full years out from my initial surgery, I had experienced some return
of sensation albeit only pain and vibratory sensation.

This brings me to another point that I think is important to
discuss at least briefly: safety. As an occupational therapist I have
taught many patients how to compensate for a lack of sensation in
their hands and feet. Decreased sensation to these areas can occur
as a result of *peripheral neuropathy* associated with some chemotherapy agents, diabetes, and several other medical conditions.
Peripheral neuropathy is basically nerve damage that occurs in the
peripheral nerves of the body. Peripheral nerves supply the skin of
the body with sensation. We typically teach patients with limited sensation in their hands and feet that they need to be more aware of
injury, heat, and cold to their extremities because their sensation is
diminished and they might not feel pain or discomfort until the
damage is already done. Similarly, if the sensation in your breasts
is as diminished as mine is, it is important to realize this and take
the necessary precautions. For example, if you lean too close to a

heat source such as a stove top, be aware that you may cause skin damage before you feel anything. If you get poked or bumped in the chest area — as I have many times — you may be tempted to just carry on without a second thought. After all, it didn't hurt a bit, right? Remember that your sensation is diminished and you may not feel pain normally in your chest area, but be sure to inspect your skin for injury. Extra care is also recommended for showering so that you avoid being scalded by hot water.

Sometimes women ask me what the implants and my overall reconstruction feel like. Typical questions are "Are they heavy?" "Can you feel them in there?" "Do you feel different?" I always welcome such questions when the asker is genuinely interested but I have a habit, perhaps due to my no-nonsense New England upbringing, of being very blunt and to the point. Depending upon my mood I might tell them that it is like wearing a plastic wrap bra 24/7. I'm joking but I'm also being 100 percent honest about how it truly feels. It is not a complaint, just a simple statement of fact. Believe me, I consider myself to be incredibly lucky to have been diagnosed with breast cancer at a time when surgical procedures are so advanced and to have access to great surgeons who used cutting-edge surgical techniques. In terms of sensation, though, if I'm sitting perfectly still, I don't feel different than I did before the surgery. But as soon as I move a little bit this way or that, or take a deep breath, I experience the foreign feeling of the reconstruction and the implants and the "Saran Wrap™ bra." In general, wearing a bra lessens this slightly alien feeling and makes me feel a little bit more held together. I also have a tendency to feel a little bit itchy, perhaps this is still the phantom sensation, and wearing the bra helps diminish this feeling as well. This is not to say that I am constantly reminded of my implants every minute of the day. In fact, I don't often stop and think about them, probably only every couple of days.

Another oddity with implant reconstruction is that your breasts may very often feel cold. At any given time I would estimate that my breasts feel about 5–10 degrees colder to the touch than the rest of my body. I have heard other women describe this temperature difference, too. And in the dead of winter, when it is really cold outside, there is a tendency for muscle spasms in the pectoralis major muscle that covers the implants. With flap procedures, however, your transplanted tissue is attached to its own blood supply so your reconstructed breasts will be the same temperature as the rest of your body.

With tissue expanders, there is the added experience and sensation associated with fills. The *fill* is when the physician gradually pumps saline into the small valve in the expander, thereby stretching the tissue in preparation for placement of a more permanent breast implant. Fills happen over a period of several months and then there is a second surgery to exchange the tissue expander for an implant. Women describe varying degrees of discomfort associated with the fill process but the description mostly involves feelings of tightness and pressure. Lisa describes her experience with fills here:

> *Fills were uncomfortable/tight but again doable. The amazing part of fills was watching your progress on a weekly basis. Positive changes were an asset with expanders and reduced much of the emotional toll I feel.*

Most women report that the feelings of tightness and discomfort after expander fills subside within 24–48 hours. Discomfort is typically managed with over-the-counter pain medications such as Tylenol™.

Exercise after Mastectomy

After mastectomy with or without reconstruction, many women will find that they have limited range of motion in their shoulders. Your arm(s) may feel tight at the shoulder and it may feel like you can't move the way you did before the surgery. If this is the case, talk to your physician about getting a referral to see a physical or occupational therapist who specializes in breast cancer and post-mastectomy rehabilitation. A few weeks out from my surgery I had some tightness in my shoulders so I did a few stretching exercises that really worked for me.

Keep in mind that as the initial healing takes place, there are going to be restrictions about how much you should be moving your arm(s). These are the *range of motion precautions* that we talked about in Chapter 2. Again, it is essential that you clearly understand these precautions before you leave the hospital. Ask about changes to these rules at each of your post-operative outpatient visits and record them in the Post-Operative Visits section at the back of this book.

Exercises can help improve the mobility and flexibility you have in your arms after surgery. Moving your affected arm also helps prevent swelling, so it is important not to guard your affected arm too much because guarding can contribute to immobility and swelling. *Guarding,* also called *protective posturing,* is when you try not to move an extremity because it hurts and you want to protect it. Sometimes people will guard after injury or surgery because the extremity is sore, not realizing that they may be doing more harm than good. When this type of protective posturing continues too long it can lead to arm swelling and/or frozen shoulder syndrome. *Frozen shoulder syndrome,* also known as *adhesive capsulitis,* is joint tightness that can occur after long-term immobility. This is discussed in more detail in the Complications section of the book.

There are some very basic things you can do early on to ensure continued mobility of your arm and to decrease the chances of developing edema, or swelling in the affected arm. The following information has been developed by the American Cancer Society in collaboration with the Oncology Section of the American Physical Therapy Association and has been adapted for the purposes of this book.

> Check with your physician *before* beginning any exercise program after your mastectomy or breast reconstruction surgery.

The Week after Surgery

The exercises listed below can be done for the first 3 to 7 days after surgery. Do not begin these exercises until your physician has given you permission.

- Use your affected arm — the arm on the side of your surgery — as you normally would when combing your hair, bathing, and eating, keeping in mind any precautions or limitations your physician has given you.

- Lie down and raise your affected arm above the level of your heart for 45 minutes. Do this two or three times a day. Put your arm on pillows so that your hand is higher than your wrist and your elbow is a little higher than your shoulder. This will help decrease the swelling that may occur after surgery.
- Exercise your affected arm while it is raised above the level of your heart by opening and closing your hand 15 to 25 times. Next, bend and straighten your elbow. Repeat this three or four times a day. This exercise helps reduce swelling by pumping lymph fluid out of your arm.
- Practice deep breathing exercises using your diaphragm at least six times a day. Lie on your back and take a slow, deep breath. Breathe in as much air as you can while trying to expand your chest and abdomen (i.e., push your belly button away from your spine). Relax and breathe out. Repeat this four or five times. This exercise will help maintain normal movement of your chest, making it easier for your lungs to work. Do deep breathing exercises often.
- Do not sleep on your affected arm or lie on that side.

Getting Started: General Guidelines

The exercises described in these pages can be done as soon as your physician gives permission. *It is very important to talk to your physician before attempting any exercises.* Here are some things to keep in mind after breast surgery:

- You will feel some tightness in your chest and armpit after surgery. This is normal and the tightness will decrease as you continue your exercises.
- Many women have burning, tingling, numbness, or soreness on the backs of the arm and/or chest wall. This is because the surgery can irritate some of your nerves. These feelings may increase a few weeks after surgery. But keep doing your exercises unless you notice unusual swelling or tenderness. If this happens, let your doctor know immediately. Sometimes rubbing or stroking the area with your hand or a soft cloth can help make the area less sensitive.

- It may be helpful to do exercises after a warm shower when muscles are warm and relaxed.

- Wear comfortable, loose clothing when doing the exercises.

- Do the exercises until you feel a slow stretch. At the end of the motion, hold the stretch and slowly count to five. It is normal to feel some pulling as you stretch the skin and muscles that have been shortened because of the surgery. Do not bounce or make any jerky movements when doing any of the exercises. You should not feel pain as you do the exercises, only gentle stretching.

- Do each exercise five to seven times. Try to do each exercise correctly. If you have trouble with the exercises, talk to your doctor. You may need to be referred to a physical or occupational therapist.

- Do the exercises twice a day until your normal flexibility and strength return. Don't overdo the number of repetitions or the frequency per day.

- Be sure to take deep breaths, breathing in and out, as you do each exercise.

- The exercises are set up so that you start them lying down, move to sitting, and finish standing up.

Exercises to Do While Lying Down

These exercises should be done on a bed or the floor. Lie down on your back with your knees and hips bent and your feet flat.

Wand Exercise

This exercise helps increase the forward motion of your shoulders. You will need a broom handle, yardstick, or other stick-like object to use as the wand in this exercise.

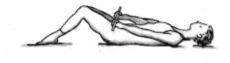

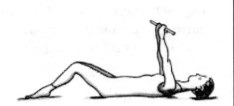

- Hold the wand in both hands with your palms facing up.
- Lift the wand up over your head as far as you can. Use your unaffected arm to help lift the wand until you feel a stretch in your affected arm.
- Hold for five seconds.
- Lower arms and repeat five to seven times.

Elbow Winging

This exercise helps increase the movement in the front of your chest and shoulder. It may take many weeks of regular exercise before your elbows will get close to the bed or floor.

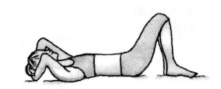

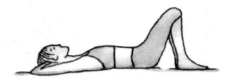

- Clasp your hands behind your neck with your elbows pointing toward the ceiling.
- Move your elbows apart and down toward the bed or floor.
- Repeat five to seven times.

Exercises to Do While Sitting Up

Shoulder Blade Stretch

This exercise helps increase your shoulder blade movement.

- Sit in a chair very close to a table with your back against the back of the chair.
- Place the unaffected arm on the table with your elbow bent and palm down. Do not move this arm during the exercise.
- Place the affected arm on the table, palm down, with your elbow straight.
- Without moving your trunk, slide the affected arm forward, toward the opposite side of the table. You should feel your shoulder blade move as you do this.
- Relax your arm and repeat five to seven times.

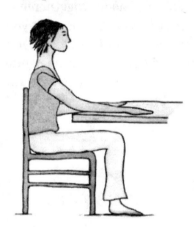

Shoulder Blade Squeeze

This exercise also helps increase shoulder blade movement.

- Facing straight ahead, sit in a chair in front of a mirror. Do not rest against the back of the chair.
- Your arms should be at your sides with your elbows bent.
- Squeeze your shoulder blades together, bringing your elbows behind you. Keep your shoulders level as you do this. Do not lift your shoulders up toward your ears.
- Return to the starting position and repeat five to seven times.

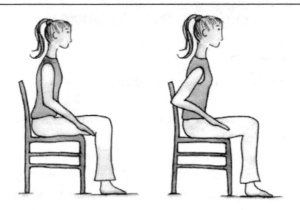

Side Bending

This exercise helps increase movement of your trunk and body.

- Sit in a chair and clasp your hands together in front of you. Lift your arms slowly over your head, straightening your arms.
- When your arms are over your head, bend your trunk to the right. Bend at your waist and keep your arms overhead.
- Return to the starting position and bend to the left.
- Repeat five to seven times.

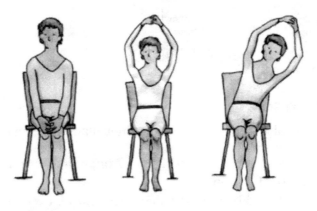

Exercises to Do While Standing

Chest Wall Stretch

This exercise helps stretch your chest.

- Stand facing a corner with your toes about eight to ten inches from the corner.
- Bend your elbows and put your forearms on the wall, one on each side of the corner. Your elbows should be as close to shoulder height as possible.
- Keep your arms and feet in place and move your chest toward the corner. You will feel a stretch across your chest and shoulders.
- Return to the starting position and repeat five to seven times.

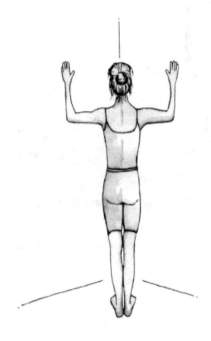

Shoulder Stretch

This exercise helps increase the mobility in your shoulder.

- Stand facing the wall with your toes about eight to ten inches from the wall.
- Put your hands on the wall. Use your fingers to "climb the wall," reaching as high as you can until you feel a stretch.
- Return to the starting position and repeat five to seven times.

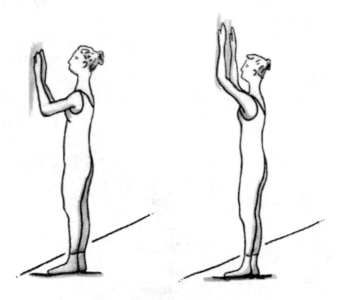

Things to Keep in Mind

Start exercising slowly and increase as you are able. Stop exercising and talk to your doctor if you:

- Get weaker, start losing your balance, or start falling
- Have pain that gets worse
- Have new heaviness in your arm
- Have unusual swelling or swelling gets worse
- Have headaches, dizziness, blurred vision, new numbness, or tingling in your arms or chest
- Don't *overdo* it. Stick with the number of repetitions recommended by your physician or therapist

It is important to exercise to keep your muscles working as well as possible, but it is also important to be safe. Talk with your doctor about the right kind of exercises for your condition, and then set goals for increasing your level of physical activity.

—Reprinted by permission of the American Cancer Society, Inc. (www.cancer.org) All Rights Reserved.

Remember to ask for a referral to a qualified occupational or physical therapist who specializes in breast cancer rehabilitation if you feel that you might need it.

There is a wonderful book called *The Breast Cancer Survivor's Fitness Plan*, written by Carolyn Kaelin, M.D., M.P.H., that outlines the various types of reconstructive surgery and the physical after-effects of each type. In the book Dr. Kaelin reviews implant, TRAM flap, and latissumus dorsi flap surgeries, and stresses the physical challenges that may develop as a result of the muscles being stretched and/or rerouted with each of these procedures. When muscles are rerouted to different areas of the body, it is only logical that other muscles will have to pick up the slack left behind. She reviews the actions of the involved muscles and explains how loss of these muscles can lead to imbalance, pain, and postural issues after surgery. She also gives specific exercises that can be done after each of these types of surgery. I think that any woman who is considering undergoing breast reconstruction should read this book to get a general idea of how the surgery is likely to impact on function.

Breast Prostheses

If you decide not to have breast reconstruction or you opt to delay your reconstruction, you may choose to wear a *breast prosthesis*. A breast prosthesis is a breast-shaped form that is worn inside a special mastectomy bra or a regular bra to provide balance and symmetry. This is a highly personal decision; many women choose to use a prosthesis while others prefer to go without. It is very important to understand, however, that in addition to the cosmetic benefits that a breast prosthesis provides, a prosthesis also provides weight and balance against the chest wall. Wearing a breast prosthesis may help avoid musculoskeletal imbalances that could result in pain and discomfort later on.

When possible, it is recommended that you meet with a certified mastectomy fitter before your surgery. If you are not sure whether or not to get a breast prosthesis, you may want to meet with a certified fitter just to get an idea about the options that are available to you. There are special camisoles and lightweight, fiber-filled breast prostheses that can be worn almost immediately after surgery. Insurance rules dictate that these products will not be covered until after the surgery. Therefore, you will need a prescription from your doctor if you want to have your breast prosthesis, mastectomy bras, or camisoles covered by insurance. In general, it is recommended that you wait six weeks after surgery before your first post-mastectomy fitting so that your skin has time to heal properly.

Your surgeon or the hospital where you are having your mastectomy may have a relationship with a certified fitter-mastectomy (CF-m) or you can use the searchable database on the American Board for Certification in Orthotics, Prosthetics, and Pedorthics (ABC) website to find someone in your area. It is important to find someone who is certified as a CF-m, which means that that person has completed educational coursework, taken a written examination, and has 500 hours of mastectomy fitting experience.

There are many mastectomy bra and prosthesis mail order companies that have certified mastectomy fitters on staff. It is strongly recommended, however, that you see a CF-m in person for your first fitting and then every year or so afterward so that you can be re-measured. Once you have found a mastectomy bra and prosthesis type that work for you, you may use the mail order companies to order additional supplies. In the beginning, however, the in-person appointment with a fitter is preferable because there is no substitute for an in-person, hands-on assessment. Besides the cosmetic reasons, there can be some real negative consequences to wearing ill-fitting mastectomy bras and breast prostheses. For example, if the weight of the prosthesis is not appropriate it can cause shoulder, back, or neck pain. You should check with your insurance company about how many bras and forms are covered and over what time period.

Here are some of the basics about prostheses, certified mastectomy fitters, and the breast prosthesis fitting process. This information is being provided with the permission of the American Board for Certification in Orthotics, Prosthetics, and Pedorthics (ABC), the governing body for credentialing certified mastectomy fitters nationwide. For more information about the ABC, or to find a fitter in your area, see their website listed in the Resources section at the back of the book.

What is a mastectomy fitter?

A mastectomy fitter is a health care professional who is specifically educated and trained in the provision of breast prostheses and post-mastectomy services. This includes patient assessment, formulation of a treatment plan, implementation of the treatment plan, follow-up, and practice management.

What is an ABC Certified Fitter-mastectomy (CF-m)?

An ABC CF-m is a health care professional who has demonstrated knowledge and competence in the field of post-mastectomy care whose qualifications have been tested and accepted by the ABC. A CF-m is also required to participate in continuing education programs to maintain certification.

What does an ABC CF-m do?

An ABC CF-m evaluates the needs and goals of the post-mastectomy patient in order to determine the appropriate prosthesis, implement a treatment plan, provide follow-up care, and coordinate these services with related medical professionals. To provide this care effectively and comprehensively, a mastectomy fitter certified by the ABC must have specialized education and skills that enable the fitter to match current and emerging prosthetic techniques and technology to the patients' needs and goals.

How can patients find an ABC CF-m?

The ABC offers a free searchable database of ABC-certified mastectomy fitters, along with a listing of ABC-accredited facilities to assist patients in finding a qualified post-mastectomy professional and facility.

What should patients look for when considering a mastectomy fitter's credentials?

A certified CF-m is required to have successfully completed the following:

- A pre-certification education course
- Written examination
- Ongoing continuing education courses

A mastectomy fitter's certification should always be verified, as this is an indication of qualifications. All mastectomy fitters certified by the ABC are bound by its standards of ethics, making them accountable to their patients/clients, physicians, and the profession.

How can patients find a facility that works best for them?

Picking the right facility is just as important as picking the right mastectomy fitter.

Patients should ask the following questions:

- *Is the facility accredited?* The ABC operates a stringent accreditation program that indicates that the facility meets strict quality guidelines. Medicare requires that all mastectomy facilities be accredited in order to receive reimbursement. Be sure to check the accreditation status of the facility you choose.
- *Does the mastectomy fitter have experience or additional training to work with different types of mastectomy prostheses?* As techniques and technology in post-mastectomy care advance, mastectomy fitters have to keep up with the changes by attending continuing education courses or

conferences. Make sure the mastectomy fitter you choose is keeping up to date.

- *How convenient is the facility?* While this might not be a final factor, patients should know that a good treatment plan will often include multiple visits, so it is helpful to consider a facility's proximity and office hours.

Before deciding on a mastectomy facility or CF-m, patients should:

- Tour the facility, meet the staff, and talk with the mastectomy fitter
- Discuss possible treatment options and get a sense of how the mastectomy fitter will approach their individual situation

What questions should a patient ask the mastectomy fitter?

- Are you certified in the provision of post-mastectomy products and services?
- Is this facility accredited by a Medicare-recognized accrediting body?
- How long will my first fitting take?
- Do you have sufficient inventory available to meet my particular needs?
- What insurances do you take?
- Will I have any out-of-pocket expenses?

How soon after surgery can a patient be fitted for a prosthesis or post-mastectomy bra?

A non-weighted form can be worn immediately after surgery. Fitting of a weighted external breast prosthesis is dependent upon proper healing after surgery. While everyone is different, the typical time frame is six to eight weeks after breast removal surgery, allowing for removal of drains, reduction of post-surgical swelling and complete healing of surgical scars.

Where are breast care services provided?

There are many different environments in which post mastectomy services are provided. The most common are post-mastectomy boutiques, a hospital cancer boutique, or a prosthetic facility. The primary concern would be to find a comfortable environment at an accredited facility with a mastectomy fitter who is certified.

Is a prescription required?
Yes, if you are seeking insurance reimbursement.

What should patients wear for a fitting?
Comfortable clothes and a blouse that is easily removed is suggested. During the fitting, privacy wraps will be provided.

What is the post-mastectomy fitting process?
The CF-m will measure and evaluate the surgical area for pressure marks, scarring, and sensitivity. The patient and fitter will discuss all appropriate treatment options including styles, shapes, and materials, as well as the patient's goals and expectations. Instructions on use and care of the items will also be provided during the fitting.

What happens if a patient's body size changes due to weight loss or weight gain?
If there is a change in condition — reduction of swelling, changes in post-surgical swelling, torso lymphedema, weight change, additional surgery or any other changes — a re-evaluation of the fit of the prosthesis, garments, and accessories is necessary.

–Reprinted with permission of the American Board for Certification in Orthotics, Prosthetics, and Pedorthics

Many of us may remember the breast prostheses that our mothers or grandmothers wore years ago. The *breast forms* and *mastectomy bras* of today bear little resemblance to those from the past. Breast forms are designed in all shapes and sizes, some with nipples and some without. Most mastectomy bras look like any other bra you might buy in a department store, except for the pocket that holds the breast form. Your CF-m will help you find a mastectomy bra and a breast form size and shape that best suits your needs.

Bras and camisoles that are worn immediately after mastectomy surgery are made of soft fabric for maximum comfort. Your first postoperative breast form will be made of a lightweight material called fiberfill. This breast form can be worn during the initial healing stages after surgery. Mastectomy camisoles will have pockets for drains. Bras may have loops for attaching drains and they will have front closures for ease of fastening and unfastening.

Foam breast forms are generally worn during the next stage of healing, before the final fittings for the silicone breast form have occurred. After six weeks or so, when the mastectomy incisions are well healed, you should make an appointment with your CF-m to determine what type of breast form is best for you. There are attachable breast forms that adhere directly to the skin and are worn under a regular bra; these forms are a good option if you have an active lifestyle. Other silicone breast forms can be worn within the pocket of a mastectomy bra. Many of the breast forms on the market today have special ventilation or moisture-absorbing features to reduce perspiration around the prosthesis.

Partial shapers are available for women who have had lumpectomy or breast reconstruction that resulted in asymmetry of the breasts. These forms will provide symmetry and balance to the breasts. They are made of soft silicone and are slightly concave on the inside so that they can accommodate the existing breast tissue. They can be worn inside a mastectomy bra or a regular bra. Swim breast forms are also available, as are specially designed swimsuits for women who have undergone mastectomy.

Externally worn silicone breast forms have a life span of about two years when properly cared for with daily cleaning. Medicare will provide one silicone breast form every two years and one non-silicone breast form every six months. Although all insurance companies will differ in their coverage, most will be in line with Medicare coverage.

Scar Management

Do not begin scar massage until your incisions are well healed and you have been cleared by your physician.

Once your incisions are well healed and your physician gives you the go-ahead, you can begin *scar massage*. The purpose of scar massage is to reduce tightness in the newly healed skin, improve blood flow to the area, and to produce a soft, supple scar. Gently massaging the tissue will also help the scar glide so that it does not adhere to the tissues underneath it. Scar tissue will continue to change for a year or more, so it is important to massage your scar continuously during this period. If you are planning to have *nipple reconstruction*, it is particularly important to perform proper scar management on the scar across your breast area to prepare the scar for the next stage of the reconstruction process. Your physician may recommend a specific type of oil or lotion be used, such as Genes Vitamin E Cream™ or Dr. E's Vitamin E Cream™.

1. Begin by putting a small amount of lotion on your fingertips.
2. Massage into the scar with the pads of your middle and index finger, using a circular motion.
3. Massage along the length of the scar and side-to-side across the scar.
4. Always begin with light pressure and gradually increase the amount of pressure over time.
5. Repeat this process one or two times per day or as instructed by your physician.
   Note: Do not massage aggressively as this may compromise skin integrity and healing.

There are many types of scar preparations on the market these days, including silicone sheeting. Products that provide ongoing light pressure tend to reduce hypertrophic-type scars. The International Advisory Panel on Scar Management suggests use of silicone gel sheeting to prevent overgrowth of scars.[25] Silicone sheeting can be costly and it does not always adhere well to skin so check with your plastic surgeon before you buy it. If you are prone to forming keloid or hypertrophic-type scars, that is, scars that tend to overgrow, be sure to mention this to your physician at the time of your initial consultation.

Exchange Surgery and Revisions

With tissue expander to implant reconstruction, also called two stage reconstruction, the temporary expander will eventually be exchanged for a more permanent implant once the optimal breast size has been achieved. With this procedure, the surgeon may form an incision in the same place as the original mastectomy scar. This exchange surgery also provides a good opportunity for the plastic surgeon to "tweak" the breast pocket in order to reposition the implant as needed to account for any asymmetries that may have occurred in the positioning of the reconstructed breasts. Because the pocket is already formed, by all accounts this surgery is much easier to recover from than the initial mastectomy and can be performed on an outpatient basis.

Many women will require revisional surgery after either implant or flap procedures in order to achieve the desired cosmetic outcome. With implant reconstruction, some possible conditions requiring revision include skin rippling, "bottoming out" of the implant, asymmetry of the implants, and *symmastia*, where the implants are too close together. Most of these conditions can be addressed through use of one or more of the following surgical techniques:

- **Lipofilling**: Use of liposuction to remove fat from one part of the body and inject it in the reconstructed breast to improve contour.
- **Reshaping the breast pocket**: Stitching the breast pocket to move the implant into desired location.
- **Use of a tissue matrix such as Alloderm**™: To provide or improve support, correct rippling, and improve overall contour of the breast.

Flap revisions may be necessary when there is poor contour of the reconstructed breast or the size of the flap is too big or small, creating aysmmetry between the breasts. As with implant procedures, problems with poor contour may be corrected with lipofilling. Asymmetries may be improved by removing a small amount of the flap, or by using liposuction or fat grafting.[26]

Most of the procedures listed here for both implant and flap revisions will take only one to two hours — longer for extensive revisions — and can be performed on an outpatient basis with twilight anesthesia. With this type of anesthesia you will be less groggy and will wake up much more quickly and easily. You should, however, have a friend or family member available to drive you home after surgery.

Nipple Reconstruction and Tattoos

An integral part of the reconstruction process is nipple reconstruction. There are several different types of nipple reconstruction and this technique, like much of the science related to breast reconstruction, is continually progressing and evolving. The skate flap, star flap, and C-V flap are all commonly used to create a nipple. The various names represent the incision shapes that are made with each type of nipple reconstruction. Sometimes the areola is formed by taking a skin graft from another part of the body such as the inner thigh. Other times, as in my situation, the areola will be outlined with a series of incisions that, once healed, will be filled in with a tattoo to provide the appropriate pigment. Some women choose to skip the entire nipple reconstruction process and go straight to the tattoo. Again, there is no right answer here. It all depends upon what you want and what will ultimately make you feel most comfortable.

Once my scars had healed and were soft and smooth, I scheduled an appointment to have my nipple reconstruction done. This procedure was done by my plastic surgeon on an outpatient basis. It was a relatively brief procedure and when I emerged from surgery I had a series of intricately formed incisions that created a circular pattern on my right breast that would ultimately become the outline for my areola. Inside that circle, my plastic surgeon used the skin of my breast to fashion a small nub, this would reconstruct the nipple. The whole area was covered in Xeroform™, which is a thin gauze that is infused with antibiotics and petroleum jelly to keep the area moist and clean. The nipple part was then covered with an oddly shaped plastic cover that would provide a bit of protection as the newly formed nipple healed. When I put on clothes, this strange little device would give what one of my fellow nipple reconstruction patient's dubbed the "fem-bot" look. Kind of a strange, robotical looking nipple outline when worn under clothes.

Several days later I returned to have my newly formed nipple and areolar complex (NAC) checked by my plastic surgeon. I remember that I brought my little daughter with me for that appointment because she was wasn't feeling well and I couldn't bring her to pre-school that day. She was only three years old at the time, very much still my baby. I'll never forget her sitting there on the end of the examination table right next to me, while the plastic surgeon unveiled my new nipple for the first time. She craned her neck around to look at the odd little nub and because she couldn't seem to grasp the word "nipple," she started calling it "Mommy's pimple." I still laugh at that sweet moment even as I write this; it reminds me that in the craziness of this whole process it important to find humor when you can.

I was instructed to wear the "fem bot" nipple protection cover (not its real name, of course) for a lot longer than I actually did. I eventually ended up with a much more flattened looking nipple than I initially had after surgery. This lack of projection is not uncommon and is described time and time again in the nipple reconstruction literature. However, the ultimate result of the nipple was perfectly satisfactory and to my liking. I returned to the plastic surgeon's office several months later for the areola tattoo. It ended up being very difficult to match the color of the dye to my existing nipple. The first time around, despite our best efforts, I ended up with sort of an orangy looking colored nipple. When I went back for a tattoo revision several months later we decided on mixing two different tones together and those colors, overlaying the previously applied tattoo, left me with a reasonably good color match of my natural nipple.

A few years ago in the FORCE conference's "Show and Tell Room" where women who have undergone mastectomies with and without reconstruction share their results with other women who are considering surgery, I saw some of the most remarkable tattoos imaginable. One of the women had undergone a flap procedure of some type and not only were her results flawless and natural looking, but her tattoos were unbelievably perfect. They were a very light brown with sort of a mottled effect that made them look completely natural.

Some women recommend going to a professional tattoo artist rather than to a plastic surgeon's office for the nipple tattoos. I considered this option briefly but when I realized that insurance wouldn't cover it and I would have to pay out of pocket, I quickly dismissed the possibility. As it was, my insurance covered the entire procedure and there was no charge for the revision. In the end, I am very happy with how my tattoo turned out. It adds a finishing touch to my breast reconstruction but, more importantly for me, having the nipple and tattoo completed allowed me to close a certain chapter of my life that was monopolized by all things cancer and mastectomy.

There are a couple of new options for women who have not yet undergone nipple reconstruction or who do not want it. A company called Reforma™ markets very life-like, prosthetic, stick-on nipples. They are reusable and self-adhering and they come in all shapes, colors, and sizes. These nipples are covered by most insurance plans.

Another option is Rub-On-Nipples™. These are temporary three dimensional nipple and areola tattoos that come in a variety of colors and are a great option for women who have undergone breast reconstruction but who have not yet undergone nipple reconstruction. They are easy to apply and last for one to two weeks before fading.

Looking in the Mirror

Before I was diagnosed with cancer I never really thought much about my breasts. For me they were always a source of anxiety more than anything else, a constant reminder of a hereditary predisposition that I was really doing my best to forget about. The day I had my drains removed was the first day that I really took a good look in the mirror to see what I looked like after the surgery. And, not surprisingly, I cried. Looking back I think it was a combination of sheer exhaustion and the news that my cancer was invasive — which I had learned only that morning — that caused me to melt into a pile of tears. The fact of the matter was that I had gotten pretty great results from my reconstructive surgery. I remember that after I looked in the mirror I went out to the living room, sat down on my husband's lap, and just started to cry. I cried because they weren't me, because for some reason I felt embarrassed, and just because. It was my release, after all that I had been through leading up to this point. It had been such a long journey and now, with chemotherapy on the horizon, it wasn't over yet. On April 10th, six days before my surgery, at about 9:30 at night my husband and I were lying in bed watching television together. A long day of work was behind us, the kids were asleep in their beds, and we were just settling down to relax with some mindless television. Something came on the television that triggered us both, at the same moment, to look at each other and say "Happy Anniversary." So much had been going on with my diagnosis and the whole process of getting ready for the mastectomy, that both of us had completely forgotten that that day was our eleventh wedding anniversary. Cancer has a tendency to come into your life like a freight train and my case was no exception, and no amount of great reconstruction was going to completely fix that or make it go away.

A few weeks after the mastectomy, once my emotions had leveled off and I was feeling better physically, I actually began to feel quite proud of my new chest. My husband, who had initially been hesitant to take a close look, was pretty delighted too! Because even though my scars hadn't really faded yet and the nipple reconstruction was not done, my breasts weren't scary or awful looking at all. In fact, they were pretty excellent. And I looked really good in clothes now and that was very important to me.

One veteran who underwent a mastectomy with tissue expander reconstruction discusses her feeling about her body after surgery:

> *I feel fine with the loss of my breasts. They were getting to be a burden with their size and gravity. I do however mourn my loss of flexibility and strength ... I am stretching and doing the prescribed exercises every day to help this along. I have a boyfriend. He has been extremely supportive, helpful, and loving through this entire ordeal top to bottom. He is excited for my new breasts and has no issues with what has changed.*

Another veteran who underwent direct to implant reconstruction writes:

> *My husband and I both like my reconstructed breasts. I had borne and nursed three kids prior to the surgery and [my breasts were] quite saggy ... cosmetically the new*

breasts are an improvement despite some scarring and rippling. No emotional effects whatsoever, once I got through the recovery period. I think it would be hard if I had another child and couldn't breastfeed, but other than that it really doesn't FEEL like I had such a radical surgery.

When a woman does not undergo breast reconstruction there is also an adjustment period. One veteran who made the decision not to reconstruct discusses her feelings:

I am just starting to come to terms with the look of no reconstruction. I was expecting to look like the photos — very thin white scars. My scars are lumpy and red but improving. I am going to have revision surgery of the scars in 6–9 months. I have some excess tissue and concavities under my armpits. The concavities will not be fixed but some recontouring will be done by removing excess tissue. My husband is not bothered by the sight of the scars and still tells me I am beautiful.

Admittedly, coming to terms with a post-mastectomy body has the potential to be a lot trickier if you are dating or not already in a committed relationship. Undertaking any new intimate relationship can be anxiety provoking for those of us who feel self-conscious about our bodies. It makes sense that this anxiety is increased when there are scars and other indicators of mastectomy or breast reconstruction that will be evident to a new partner. There are several books that address the topics of body image, sexuality, and partner reaction after mastectomy included in the Resources section at the back of this book.

Rehabilitation after Breast Surgery: Questions and Answers with Sara Cohen, OTR/L, CLT-LANA

Sara Cohen is a registered occupational therapist with more than fifteen years of experience specializing in the treatment of women with breast cancer. She is employed by Memorial Sloan-Kettering

Cancer Center at the Evelyn H. Lauder Breast Center in New York City. Sara is a Certified Lymphedema Therapist. In this section, Sara answers some of the most common questions women may ask after breast surgery.

What are some of the conditions that would require the services of a physical therapist or occupational therapist following treatment for breast cancer? How common are these conditions?

Surgery, chemotherapy, radiation therapy, and hormonal therapy all have side effects. Each woman responds differently, depending upon the type of treatment she receives, and how her body is affected by the treatment. Some women recover quickly with limited physical side effects, and others have ongoing physical problems. Many women report cognitive and emotional difficulties following treatment for breast cancer, as well as fatigue during and after chemotherapy and radiation therapy.

It is important to note that after your surgery, you will have symptoms that do not require a visit with a rehab professional. It is normal to have mild swelling after surgery, and this will usually go away by itself. After surgery, many women report altered sensations in their armpits or upper arms, such as tenderness, tightness, numbness and tingling, pins and needles, burning, or a feeling of water running down their arm or side. These are also normal, and will slowly disappear as your body heals. It may take a year or more for the sensations to fade.

One side effect of breast cancer surgery that many women have heard or read about is a condition called lymphedema. Lymphedema is a chronic swelling that can appear in the hand, arm, breast, or chest wall on the side where lymph nodes were removed. If you had a procedure called sentinel lymph node biopsy, your risk of developing lymphedema is very low; as little as seven percent of people who have this surgery develop lymphedema.[27] If you had a procedure called axillary lymph node dissection, your risk of developing lymphedema is higher. Up to thirty percent of women develop lymphedema following this surgery.[28] If you develop lymphedema, you should contact a Certified Lymphedema Therapist (CLT) for an evaluation. Both occupational therapists and physical therapists can be CLTs, but they must have special training to earn this designation.

Another common side effect is called *cording*, or *axillary web syndrome*. Women often notice a string or cord that appears in the armpit, and extends down the arm to the elbow and even to the wrist and hand. This cord can cause pain, tightness, and limited movement of the shoulder, elbow, and wrist. Sometimes the cord will go away by itself. However, if symptoms persist, you should seek treatment. Both occupational therapists and physical therapists can treat this condition.

Other breast cancer-related physical conditions that can be treated by a physical therapist or an occupational therapist include:

▪ Tendonitis of the shoulder and "frozen shoulder," which can happen if you don't exercise sufficiently after your surgery. Studies show that people who had breast cancer surgery are more at risk for these problems.
▪ Neuropathy (tingling and numbness), which can be a side effect of certain chemotherapies

Many women report cognitive difficulties during and after treatment for breast cancer. The phrase "chemo brain" is a term coined by patients who report difficulty with memory and word finding, concentration, and organizing their time. Some women also experience anxiety, depression, as well as changes in their self-esteem. Fatigue is a common side effect of treatment for breast cancer. These problems can affect all areas of life, including basic self-care (for example, brushing your hair), job functions, leisure activities, and social activities. Occupational therapists have training in helping women overcome and compensate for these problems.

How do I know what type of therapist I need? How do physical therapists and occupational therapists differ when it comes to post-breast cancer rehabilitation?

Physical therapists are health care professionals who use treatment techniques to help promote the ability to move, reduce pain, restore function, and prevent disability (http://www.apta.org). Occupational therapists are health care professionals who modify activities and environments to help people participate in their everyday activities or occupations, such as self-care, work, leisure, and social activities (http://www.aota.org).

When it comes to post-breast cancer rehabilitation, both occupational therapists and physical therapists can address common side effects. While there is some overlap in their services, there are some differences as well. For example, both occupational and physical therapists have received extensive training in anatomy and physiology, and can be certified as lymphedema therapists. As a result, both physical therapists and occupational therapists use exercise and other physical techniques to treat problems with shoulder mobility, cording, and lymphedema.

On the other hand, physical therapists and occupational therapists have a different approach to treatment. Physical therapy evaluation and treatment focuses on your physical difficulties. Physical therapists may use exercise, hands-on techniques, and treatments such as heat or ultrasound to help improve your physical fitness and health. Occupational therapy evaluation and treatment looks at your physical challenges and also considers any cognitive and emotional difficulties that can interfere with your daily life. By breaking down your activities into smaller pieces, occupational therapists can then suggest specific exercises to help improve your function and resume these activities. They may also teach you how to conserve energy and modify activities when you are fatigued, or teach you how to combat difficulties with memory and concentration.

What are the criteria for needing rehabilitation services after breast surgery? How soon after surgery should I consider consulting with a rehabilitation professional?

Tell your doctor or nurse about any physical, cognitive, or functional difficulties that develop so he or she can determine if you should be treated by a physical therapist or occupational therapist. Some temporary swelling and arm symptoms are common after breast cancer surgery. Your medical team should help you understand what is normal and what is not, and how long temporary symptoms will last. You should be referred to a physical therapist or occupational therapist if the symptoms continue beyond what is considered normal or are interfering with your daily activities.

Studies show that it is important to do gentle exercise following surgery for breast cancer. If your medical team does not show you some basic exercises, you should ask for a consultation with a physical therapist or occupational therapist so that you can learn how to safely regain the mobility and strength in your arm.

How often and for how long does one typically see a therapist?
The physical therapist or occupational therapist will develop an individual treatment plan for you. Some plans may require only one or two visits. Other plans might require that you see the therapist several times per week in order to receive the most benefit from therapy. Generally, physical therapists and occupational therapists are covered by insurance, although some insurance companies have limits on the amount or type of therapy you can receive. Insurance will pay for the therapy as long as you are making progress. Once you are no longer improving, the therapist will instruct you in a home management program. You will need to continue this program on your own, or with the help and support of friends or family.

You should be aware that some side effects of breast cancer treatment are temporary. Other side effect may continue for a long time, or may be permanent. It is difficult for many patients to accept that their bodies are different. They want to forget about the cancer and return to their pre-cancer lives. Rehabilitation professionals can help reduce the risk of ongoing problems, but they cannot fix everything. It helps to have an open mind and to talk with your therapist about the problems that are of most concern to you.

What activities should I avoid while I am undergoing therapy?
Ask your occupational therapist or physical therapist to tell you about any precautions to take while undergoing therapy.

Is it advisable to undergo other therapies, such as massage or acupuncture at the same time, or will they interfere with physical therapy or occupational therapy?
What is most important is that all of the members of your health care team have a full understanding of your treatment plan. If you are seeing a physical therapist or occupational therapist, be sure to let your therapist know about any other therapies that you are currently receiving or planning to receive. This includes medical treatments such as chemotherapy, hormonal therapy, radiation therapy, as well as complementary therapies such as acupuncture and massage. Your therapist will let you know if there is anything you should avoid while receiving physical therapy or occupational therapy.

What things can I do on my own to ensure the success of my rehabilitation?

The most important ingredient in the success of your rehabilitation program is communicating with your therapist. If you are not clear about the therapist's instructions, you must let the therapist know. If you are unable to follow the therapist's recommendations, it is vital that you inform the therapist so that together, you can alter the plan. Do not be embarrassed to honestly report how you are doing with your "homework." The therapist cannot help you if he or she is unaware of what you have been doing in working toward your goals at home.

How do I find a therapist who has specialized knowledge about post-breast cancer therapy? How do I know a therapist has this knowledge/experience?

Word of mouth is one way to find a good therapist. Another way is to ask your doctor for a recommendation. You can also call your local hospital rehabilitation department to find out if they have an outpatient rehabilitation program. When speaking with a potential therapist, you should feel free to ask how frequently he or she treats post-breast cancer patients. You may want to pick someone who has more experience. In addition, many therapists take classes beyond school to better understand the needs of women who have been treated for breast cancer. You can ask the therapist if she has taken any courses relating to post-breast cancer rehabilitation. Therapists who have received special training in the management of lymphedema may have the credentials CLT (Certified Lymphedema Therapist) after their physical therapist and occupational therapist license. You can contact the National Lymphedema Network for help in finding a CLT near you (www.lymphnet.org).

I'm trying to decide what type of breast reconstruction would be best for me. Can you tell me how my recovery process might differ if I choose no reconstruction, implants, or a flap procedure?

Deciding whether to have reconstruction, or what kind to have, is a complicated process. Not every woman will be a candidate for the different kinds of reconstruction surgery. This is based on your body type and your past surgical history. There are psychological and social effects of the decision as well. You should talk with your medical team or a nurse or social worker to help you make this decision.

The two main types of reconstruction are breast implants and flap procedures. Some women have a combination of the two procedures. With an implant, you may first have a tissue expander placed in your chest. The expander will be slowly inflated over six to eight weeks. At a later date, depending upon your situation, the expander will be replaced with the permanent implant. Another type of implant surgery is direct to implant surgery. With this type of surgery, the implant is placed immediately after the mastectomy and a pocket is formed with a tissue matrix to keep the implant in place. In the flap procedure, tissue from another part of your body is moved to your chest to create a new breast. There are a number of kinds of flap procedures. The recovery time from a flap procedure is longer than for an implant procedure. There are pros and cons to every procedure. You should discuss with your surgeon the best option for you.

If you do not have reconstruction surgery, you will be allowed to move your arm above your head and behind your back sooner than if you do have reconstruction. If you have reconstruction surgery, your body will require more time to heal, and you will have certain precautions about the type of exercise you are allowed to do. You should talk with your nurse or surgeon for details about which exercises are right for you.

I had a few lymph nodes removed on both sides at the time of my bilateral mastectomy. Am I at risk for lymphedema? Should I avoid blood draws and needlesticks in both arms?
If you had any lymph nodes removed from your armpit, you are at risk for lymphedema. Your risk depends upon the type of surgery that you had. If you had a sentinel lymph node biopsy, your risk of developing lymphedema is very low. If you had an axillary lymph node dissection, your risk is higher. Because the risk with sentinel lymph node biopsy is very low, some doctors allow blood draws and needle sticks following this procedure. There is some controversy within the lymphedema community about this recommendation. Some continue to recommend using an alternative location, such as a leg or foot. Speak with your doctor to help decide what is best for you.

If you notice swelling or have signs of lymphedema in either arm, then you should avoid using that arm for blood draws and needle sticks. You should also consult with a lymphedema therapist to set up a treatment plan.

What is the treatment for lymphedema?
Treatment for lymphedema can be simple or intensive. A trained lymphedema therapist can help you choose the best program for you.

Treatment has four main components:

- *Instruction in skin care*: For more details, see the skin care precautions from the National Lymphedema Network that are listed in the next section of this book.
- *Compression*: Compression helps prevent fluid from building up in the tissue. It can be applied in the form of an elastic garment, low-stretch bandages, or other types of compression devices.
- *Exercise*: An exercise program helps to stimulate the lymph vessels. It is important to increase the amount of exercise slowly, so that you do not overwhelm the lymph vessels.
- *Massage*: A gentle form of massage called manual lymphatic drainage (MLD) is recommended. Vigorous massage may provoke fluid production. Lymphatic massage helps the body move the fluid to alternate drainage areas that have not been affected by your breast surgery.

You should work with your therapist to set up a treatment plan that is right for you. The plan should take into account your lifestyle and preferences. It takes time to figure out the best plan to keep the swelling under control. Talk with your therapist about any problems you have with your treatment. Your therapist can help you change your plan so it works better for you.

Lymphedema Prevention

As mentioned, after removal of lymph nodes, through *sentinel lymph node biopsy* or *axillary lymph node dissection*, there is a possibility of developing lymphedema. The lymphatic system is composed of a series of vessels and lymph nodes that carry a watery fluid called *lymph* throughout the body. Lymphedema is a swelling that can occur in the chest or arm when the flow of the lymphatic system is impaired or interrupted after mastectomy. If left untreated, over time lymphedema can become chronic and more difficult to treat, and can affect your ability to use your arm for daily activities.

Before surgery, it is important that baseline measurements are taken on both of your arms. Ask your nurse or physician about this and make careful note of where the measurements are taken. When follow-up measurements are taken at a later date they need to be done at exactly the same location so that the measurements are accurate.

Immediately after surgery, you should be given a lymphedema alert bracelet or some type of identifier to wear on your affected arm(s) to indicate to hospital staff that needle sticks and blood pressure readings should not be taken on that arm. It should also be clearly posted above your hospital bed that there should be "no blood draws or blood pressures" taken in your affected arm. It is important that you and your family members are aware of this precaution so that you can remind staff during your hospital stay.

Warning Signs of Lymphedema

The warning signs of lymphedema as outlined by the National Lymphedema Network include:

- A sensation of fullness in the limb(s).
- Skin feeling tight, decreased flexibility in the hand or wrist.
- Difficulty fitting into clothing in one specific area, or ring, wristwatch, bracelet tightness.
- If you notice persistent swelling, it is very important that you seek immediate medical advice and get at least one second opinion. Early diagnosis and treatment improves both the prognosis and the condition.

—Reprinted from the NLN Website by Saskia Thiadens, RN, with permission from the National Lymphedema Network, Inc.

There are a number of strategies that the National Lymphedema Network recommends to help prevent lymphedema from developing. Because lymphedema can develop at any time in a patient's lifetime following lymph node injury or removal, it is recommended that these precautions be taken on an ongoing basis. Compression garments can be used as both a preventive and treatment measure when properly fitted by a Certified Lymphedema Therapist (CLT).

Lymphedema Risk Reduction Practices

I. Avoid trauma/injury to the skin to reduce risk of infection.

- Keep extremity clean and dry.
- Apply moisturizer daily to prevent chapping or chafing of skin.
- Give attention to nail care; do not cut cuticles.
- Protect exposed skin with sunscreen and insect repellent.
- Use care with razors to avoid nicks and skin irritation.
- If possible, avoid punctures such as injections and blood draws.
- Wear gloves while doing activities that may cause skin injury (i.e., washing dishes, gardening, working with tools, using chemicals such as detergent).
- If scratches or punctures to skin occur, wash with soap and water, apply antibiotics, and observe for signs of infection such as redness.
- If a rash, itching, redness, pain, increased skin temperature, fever or flu-like symptoms occur, contact your physician immediately for early treatment of possible infection.

Activity/Lifestyle

- Gradually build up the duration and intensity of any activity or exercise.
- Take frequent rest periods during activity to allow for limb recovery.

- Monitor the extremity during and after activity for any change in size, shape, tissue, texture, soreness, heaviness, or firmness.
- Maintain an optimal weight.

Avoid Limb Constriction

- If possible, avoid having blood pressure taken on the at-risk extremity.
- Wear loose fitting jewelry and clothing.

Compression Garments

- Should be well-fitting.
- Support the at-risk limb with a compression garment during strenuous activity (i.e., weight lifting, prolonged standing, running) except in patients with open wounds or with poor circulation in the at-risk limb.
- Consider wearing a well-fitting compression garment for air travel.

Extremes of Temperature

- Avoid exposure to extreme cold, which can be associated with rebound swelling or chapping of skin.
- Avoid prolonged (greater than 15 minutes) exposure to heat, particularly hot tubs and saunas.
- Avoid placing limb in water temperatures above 102° Fahrenheit (38.9° Celsius).

—Reprinted from the NLN Website by Saskia Thiadens, RN, with permission from the National Lymphedema Network, Inc.

A couple of years ago I was lucky enough to attend a lecture given by Kathryn Schmitz, PhD, MPH, when she spoke at one of the FORCE conferences. You will remember that FORCE is an organization that is dedicated to providing support and education to women who are at risk for hereditary breast and ovarian cancers.

Dr. Schmitz talked about the research she had been doing with the Physical Activity and Lymphedema Trial at the University of Pennsylvania. In this study, women who were at risk for developing breast cancer–related lymphedema were enrolled in a program of slow, progressive, and supervised weight lifting that took place over the course of one year. The findings of this study upended much of the traditional wisdom and advice that has been given for years about using the affected arm after mastectomy for lifting. An excerpt from Dr. Schmitz's results indicates that:

> *Contrary to common guidelines to avoid lifting with the affected limb, we found that weight lifting did not significantly affect the severity of breast cancer–associated lymphedema.... In addition, weight lifting reduced the number and severity of arm and hand symptoms, increased muscular strength, and reduced the incidence of lymphedema exacerbations as assessed by a lymphedema specialist.*[29]

In other words, it appears that women who are at risk of developing lymphedema after a breast cancer diagnosis may actually be helped and not, as was once believed, harmed by weight-lifting types of activities provided these activities are undertaken in a slow, progressive manner. The results of this study are helping to change the way experts think and the way they educate their patients about exercise and lymphedema.

The National Lymphedema Network has released a "position paper" outlining considerations for air travel in patients who have known lymphedema or may be at risk for developing lymphedema. It is believed that the "diminished pressure in the airplane cabin will result in a decrease in the fluid moved in to the lymphatic system,"[30] thereby increasing the possibility of a lymphedema flare up. Compression garments during air travel are recommended for individuals with known lymphedema. It is recommended that individuals who are deemed to be "at risk" for lymphedema "... take precautions when flying and should consider compression to the affected limb."[31] Individuals who are considered to be at risk include those who have had lymph nodes removed or who have undergone radiation treatments.

If lymphedema develops or if you want to find out more about compression garments for air travel, be sure to ask your physician to refer you to a Certified Lymphedema Therapist (CLT). Both the National Lymphedema Network and the Lymphology Association of North America websites, listed at the back of this book, are good resources for finding credentialed therapists in your area.

Complications

As with any type of surgery, things occasionally can go wrong during the healing process. With any luck at all, you will never have to refer to this section of the book. But on the off chance that you do, I want to outline some of the most basic complications associated with mastectomy and breast reconstruction so that you can have some idea of what you are dealing with. Some of the most common complications include infection, frozen shoulder syndrome, capsular contracture, rupture or deflation of implants, poor wound healing, axillary web syndrome, and pain.

Infection

Infection is one of the biggest concerns after surgery of any kind. There are a few steps that you can take to prevent infections.

- **Use antibacterial soap**: Bathe carefully with antibacterial soap the night or morning *before* your surgery.
- **Take antibiotics**: You will be sent home with a prescription for an antibiotic. You must take the medication religiously and until completely finished as instructed by your physician.
- **Wash hands often**: You should practice impeccable hand washing with antibacterial soap before handling your drains or performing any wound care.
- **Bathing**: Do not take a bath if your drains are still in place or if you have open wounds. Shower *only* when you have been given the go ahead by your physician.

▪ **Never clean inside your drains**: This is a very dangerous practice; it can introduce bacteria into the drain system and can lead to serious and life-threatening infection.

▪ **Care givers:** Ask your physician, nurse, and care giver to wash his or her hands and/or to wear gloves.

Sometimes despite our best preventive efforts, infection develops anyway. There may be absolutely nothing that you could have done better or differently to avoid the infection. If you have had surgery with implants or expanders, one of the possible outcomes of infection is that the tissue expander or implant may need to be removed so that proper wound healing can occur. Perhaps several months later, once your infection has completely resolved, the expander or implant may be replaced. Possible treatments for infection include drainage of fluid, treatment with IV antibiotics, and *debridement* of tissue. Debridement is when dead tissue is carefully removed to promote better wound healing.

After all that you have already been through, loss of an expander or implant can be a devastating development. Some women who experience repeated implant failure will eventually opt to undergo flap procedures.

Frozen Shoulder/Adhesive Capsulitis

Frozen shoulder syndrome or *adhesive capsulitis* is a condition that sometimes develops after mastectomy. Frozen shoulder develops after mastectomy because of:

> ... *severely limiting your range of motion in your shoulder and arm for a prolonged time after surgery. Tightness in the joint results and worsens until normal movements become acutely painful.*[32]

In the exercise section, I talked about how *protective posturing*, also known as *guarding*, can lead to complications like frozen shoulder syndrome. Due to the lack of mobility, a shortening and tightening of the structures surrounding the shoulder joint occur resulting in decreased mobility. Radiation treatments can also contribute to these types of tissue changes. During occupational therapy training, one of my professors told us "motion is lotion." In other words, when you move a joint — even if there is some mild discomfort with the movement — you are actually helping to loosen it up and increase mobility. If you continuously keep your shoulder in a fixed position, as happens with guarding, you are simply contributing to a vicious cycle of immobility.

If you think you may already have frozen shoulder syndrome or feel you are at risk for developing it, you should ask your physician to give you a referral to see an occupational therapist or a physical therapist. This professional will most likely use a combination of heat, gentle stretching, and therapeutic exercise to help you regain the previous range of motion in your affected arm. To prevent frozen shoulder syndrome from developing, you should continue to move your arm as you normally would when doing basic self-care activities such as brushing teeth, combing hair, and dressing. Remember to follow any post-surgical precautions regarding movement and lifting and try to move your arm safely within these limits.

Capsular Contracture

Capsular contracture is a complication that occurs when a thickened pocket of scar tissue forms around a breast implant. If the scar tissue begins to tighten too much, it will start to squeeze the implant causing hardening or deformity of the breast. If you imagine squeezing a water balloon in the cup of your hand you can get an idea of what capsular contracture is like. The breast pocket that surrounds the implant is like the cup of your hand. When your hand is relaxed it gently cups the balloon leaving it with a smooth, rounded appearance. If you squeeze the balloon, the nice smooth, rounded appearance of the balloon can bulge and become deformed. When this happens with your implant, you may have a very tight-feeling breast that is not symmetrical with your other breast. There is a grading system for capsular contracture called the Baker Grading System. Grades III and IV may require a revision surgery called *capsulectomy*. A capsulectomy is when the surgeon breaks up and removes the scar tissue surrounding the implant. With this surgery, however, there is no guarantee that the deforming scar tissue will not form again. The use of an acellular dermis in reconstruction may prevent capsular contracture.

The Baker Grading System is as follows:

Grade I	Breast is normally soft and looks natural.
Grade II	Breast is a little firm but looks normal.
Grade III	Breast is firm and looks abnormal.
Grade IV	Breast is hard, painful, and looks abnormal.

—Reprinted with permission from the FDA. [33]

You may be able to avoid capsular contracture by performing regular breast massage to keep the implant mobilized within its pocket. Regular breast massage will help push the boundaries of the pocket, preventing it from shrinking too much and thus causing capsular contracture. As of this writing, the American Society of Plastic Surgeons does not endorse a particular protocol for massaging implants after breast reconstruction. Check with your plastic surgeon about what he or she recommends regarding massaging implants and be sure to get clearance from your physician before you begin massaging your implants.

Rupture and Deflation of Breast Implants

Breast implants are continuously improving as technology advances, however, they are still prone to rupture and deflation. Rupture and deflation occur when the outer shell of the implant is damaged and the inner contents leak out of the shell. The following information is reprinted with permission from the FDA.

Some possible reasons for rupture/deflation of breast implants include[34]:

■ Normal aging of the implant
■ Damage by surgical instruments

- Too much handling during surgery
- Damage by procedures to the breast, such as biopsies and fluid drainage
- Compression during mammographic imaging
- Stresses such as trauma or intense physical pressure
- Capsular contracture
- Overfilling or underfilling of saline-filled breast implants

Doctors usually recommend removal of the implant if it has ruptured, regardless of whether it is saline-filled or silicone gel-filled.

Rupture/Deflation of Saline-Filled Breast Implants

Saline-filled breast implants rupture/deflate when the saline solution leaks either through an unsealed or damaged valve, or through a break in the implant shell. Implant deflation usually happens immediately but sometimes may happen slowly over a period of days. Deflation of saline-filled breast implants is noticed by a loss of size or shape of the implant.
    —*Reprinted from the FDA.*[35]

Rupture/Deflation of Silicone Implants

Unlike rupture or deflation of a saline breast implant, when a silicone implant ruptures it might not be immediately noticeable. The silicone gel may stay within the breast's scar capsule. In this case, the rupture can be best diagnosed through MRI.[35]

There is a new generation of implants called *cohesive gel implants* or *gummy bear implants*. With a texture and feel much like gummy bear candy, the inner material in this type of implant is soft solid silicone, not liquid. As the name indicates, the implant is made up entirely of a cohesive gel so if the implant sustains damage, liquid may not leak into the body. These new implants are available on a limited basis through a select group of physicians who have agreed to participate in "after market" studies. They are not FDA approved as of this writing.

Post-Mastectomy Pain Syndrome

Post-mastectomy pain syndrome is a chronic pain condition that sometimes develops after mastectomy or lumpectomy surgery. The pain may be associated with damage to the intercostobrachial nerve[36] and is generally thought to be a type of pain called *neuropathic pain*, a chronic pain condition that occurs after some type of injury to the nervous system. The pain may be located in the underarm, arm, shoulder, or chest wall and it is often described as a "burning" or "shooting" pain. Some mastectomy veterans call these pains "lightening bolts." Incidence of post-mastectomy pain syndrome is believed to be much higher following axillary lymph node dissection.[37] The pain can develop immediately after surgery or, in some cases, years later. Neuropathic pain syndromes are notoriously difficult to treat but some treatment possibilities you can discuss with your doctor include the use of non-steroidal anti-inflammatory medications, nerve block injections, myofascial release, desensitization, physical therapy, and acupuncture.[38] The use of anti-depressants has also been an effective treatment for some neuropathic pain.[39] If your pain is becoming chronic, you should consider seeing a physician who specializes in pain management and has treated other patients with post-mastectomy pain syndrome.

Axillary Web Syndrome

Axillary web syndrome can occur when there is damage or interruption to the lymph nodes as with sentinel or axillary lymph node dissection. Symptoms of axillary web syndrome include tightness, limited range of motion, pain, and webbing or "cording" in the underarm, elbow, and/or thumb.[40] Axillary web syndrome can occur anytime after surgery but is most likely to present in the first eight weeks after surgery.[41]Axillary web syndrome is thought to be the result of blockages in the veins and lymphatic system, and can also be related to increased scar tissue.[42]

The lymphedema education organization Step Up, Speak Out recommends that patient's undertake limited stretching of the arm during the immediate post-operative period in order to ensure that the delicate structures making up the lymaphatic system have time to heal,[43] thereby reducing the risk of developing axillary web syndrome later.

Axillary web sydrome can often be treated successfully by an occupational therapist or physical therapist who is experienced in treating post-mastectomy patients. Treatment techniques include gentle stretching and scar release. If you have been diagnosed with axillary web syndrome, ask your physician for a referral to a qualified therapist.

Poor Wound Healing

Poor wound healing occurs when wounds fail to heal at a typical rate. Some reasons for delayed wound healing include recent chemotherapy, infection, seroma, hematoma, history of smoking, previously radiated skin, compromised nutritional status, and decreased circulation to the wound. The Breastcancer.org website, which is a great resource for all things related to breast cancer and mastectomy, outlines a number of tips for promoting good wound healing,[20] including:

- **Hand washing:** Be fastidious with your hand washing routine before and after performing any wound care. Use an antibacterial hand soap and warm water, and remember to clean under your fingernails. Make sure any health care provider who treats your wound also washes his or her hands and wears examination gloves.
- **Dressings:** When you remove used dressings, be very careful with pulling off adhesives, gauze, and bandages. If the wound is oozing, the gauze bandage may become stuck to the wound. Use extreme care in removing the gauze so as not to reopen the wound.
- **Wound care:** Clean the wound every day using whatever cleanser your physician has recommended. Saline is often used if there is no infection. Do not scrub the wound or attempt to remove scabs. Pat the wound dry with clean gauze.
- **Use new bandages and dressings:** This is common sense. Sterile, individually wrapped, gauze and bandages should always be used.
- **Nutrition:** Eat a diet that is rich in protein and Vitamins A and C. Foods that are rich in Vitamin A include carrots, leafy green vegetables, butternut squash, dried apricots, and cantaloupe. Foods that are rich in Vitamin C include broccoli, cauliflower, leafy

greens, oranges, strawberries, kiwi, and bell peppers. Good sources of protein are beans, lean meats, poultry, lentils, peanuts, hard cheeses, and fish such as tuna, salmon, and halibut.

Going Back to Work

When you are cleared to return to work after mastectomy will depend upon what type of work you do and what type of procedure you underwent. In general, after mastectomy with no reconstruction you will probably be ready to return to work much earlier than if you had reconstruction. That said, if your work is very physical in nature, you may want to delay your return to work a bit longer. When I was first diagnosed with breast cancer I was working as a pediatric occupational therapist for small children, up to age five. This involved a lot of work with a large therapy ball that required me to have a fair amount of upper body strength in order to support their body weight. I had decided I was going to take six weeks off from my job and my physicians went along with that plan. Ultimately, because I went on to do chemotherapy, I took six months off and was well healed by the time I returned to work.

This mastectomy veteran describes her experience going back to work after direct to implant reconstruction:

> *I returned to work almost three weeks after the surgery. For me it was too soon, I did have significant pain and it wasn't well controlled and I was still tired at the time. My job isn't physical but I have a long commute. I would say one more week would have made a big difference and I would have waited four weeks if I had to do it over again.*

Lisa underwent prophylactic mastectomy with tissue expanders and eventual implant placement. She describes her experience returning to work and gives advice here:

> *At exactly five weeks post-prophylactic mastectomy/ expanders I returned to work full time. I do not recommend full-time work until at least four weeks. Fatigue is the biggest reason for not returning sooner. Know your body and listen to it as well.*

Kim also underwent mastectomy with tissue expander placement; at two weeks post-op she reports:

> *I'm definitely not ready yet. I'm due back in two weeks, a total of one month out. I am hoping to be in full swing by then, my employer will not allow me to come back until I can fit my job description 100 percent, which does include lifting at least 40 pounds. So far, I've been recovering well from what I can tell and hope to return on schedule.*

Debra had a mastectomy with flap reconstruction. She reports that she returned to work after four weeks but notes:

> *... it was too soon. Go back in eight weeks. Take your time. Don't rush it. Give your body a chance to heal.*

Be sure to get clearance from your physician before returning to work. This is particularly important if you are going to be expected to do physical work that requires a lot of lifting, bending, or twisting. And remember that even sitting at a desk all day can be exhausting. If your employer will allow it, you may want to return to work for half days or just a couple of days a week until you are feeling stronger. Also remember that if you have had any type of complication, this may set your schedule back a few weeks.

If you are a stay-at-home mom, the challenge for you is to make sure that you are not overdoing it too soon. One stay-at-home mom I surveyed responded that she had help for four weeks after surgery. If you have family that can pitch in or you can swing it financially to hire someone to help, I think this is good advice. When we are at home, our kids — despite our condition — have a tendency to think we are "on call." It is important that you don't lift your children too soon or perform any other activities that will jeopardize your recovery. Amanda is a stay at home mom who underwent mastectomy with tissue expanders, she reports:

> *I was able to lift them after three weeks. I was still pretty exhausted the first couple of weeks post-op, so I would recommend at least 3–4 weeks off.*

Again, make sure your physician is on board with your timetable for returning to full-time "Mom" status. And make sure he or she understands what that means for you in terms of lifting children, pushing strollers and grocery carts, doing housework, etc.

Clinical Follow-up after Mastectomy

One thing you may have gathered in the process of reading this book is that there is very little within the realm of mastectomy recovery that is engraved in stone. This is also true with clinical follow-up care after mastectomy. Most physicians recommend a clinical breast exam once or twice a year but the recommendations for ultrasound, MRI, and so on vary greatly. My surgical oncologist recommends that I come to see him twice yearly for clinical breast exams. I am also expected to follow-up with my medical oncologist on a regular basis to have my blood drawn. I try to coordinate these appointments so that I am being seen by one of them every three months or so. About one year after my mastectomy I was sent for an MRI to assess the integrity of the implant and make sure there were no "hot spots" in the small amount of remaining breast tissue. Since that time, no further imaging has been recommended. Many of the women I have spoken with are recommended to have a yearly MRI or ultrasound on the affected side but again, this ultimately depends upon what your doctor feels is necessary. And, of course, it goes without saying that if you have had a unilateral mastectomy, the unaffected breast should still be followed up with self-exam, clinical breast exam, and regular mammograms and imaging as directed by your physician. If you discover a lump or any irregularities on either your affected or unaffected breast you should see your physician as soon as possible.

4

Voices

A funny thing happened while I was writing this book, something that I honestly hadn't expected. When I sent the first draft of Chapter 1 to my editor for review, she sent me back lots of comments, including one that said: "How do you prepare yourself emotionally for this?" She was right, I had barely talked about the emotional process at all. And I suppose, after thinking about it for a while, I decided that what she was asking is the hardest question of all to answer.

By that point I had established a core team of mastectomy veterans, all FORCE women, who had completed my online survey and then emailed me privately to express their willingness to participate further in the book. So I naively set about asking them to share with me how they prepared emotionally to undergo mastectomy. Essentially, I was asking them to share some of their deepest, most intimate thoughts and feelings with me. But at the time that hadn't occurred to me. I sent that first email with a bunch of questions about the emotional process and then I waited for responses to flood into my in-box ... and I waited. Days passed and not a single response from the ten or so women who I had e-mailed. I decided that I had crossed a line and had asked too much of them. I had pushed too far and pried into their private lives, thoughts, and feelings.

And then one day I had a response in my mailbox; it was from Sue. And then a couple of days later I had another response, this time from Laurie. Slowly, over the course of the next few weeks, more and more responses filtered into my mailbox. As I read the responses I was overwhelmed by the "story" that each woman told and the strength and courage they showed in their unique, individual circumstances, all of them choosing mastectomy for personal and health reasons. I was moved by the decisions they had made, the heartaches they had endured watching other family members suffer, and the courage that each one of them showed in going forward. The thoughts and feelings they had entrusted to me left me with a deep sense of responsibility — a responsibility to write the best book I could write and to help share these voices so that women who find themselves in similar situations will know that they are not alone. Someday, when all is said and done, and this book is written, I hope to be able to meet each and every one of these women in person and give them a big hug.

This is a part of the book that I never intended to write. And now, as it turns out, it is my favorite part of the entire book. I love it and I am moved by each one of the stories from these beautiful women every time I read them. As you read the stories of these women you may be able to relate to their stories. They may be the same age as you, have a family history like yours, or something in their story might just strike a chord. Most of all, I hope that their stories will inspire you and help you feel as though you are not alone on this journey.

Linda, Age 45

I am Amy's older sister, a co-author and a cancer previvor.

We have a very strong family history of breast cancer. As a nurse, I knew that my sisters and I were at heightened risk for breast cancer, too. Surveillance became a part of my life early on. I began with my baseline mammogram at age 29 (approximately ten years prior to the youngest family member's age of diagnosis) and yearly clinical breast exams as well as sporadic self-breast exams. When I was in my late 30s I started having abnormal nipple discharge. I had some testing done that showed atypical ductal cells. As a nurse practitioner I was well aware of my heightened breast cancer risk level with family history alone, but now this test result gave me reason for further concern. I consulted several breast specialists and my options were laid out: 1) continue surveillance (diagnostic mammograms and ultrasounds and alternating MRI every six months) and then consider starting chemoprevention, such as Tamoxifen, at age 40 if I was done with childbearing, or 2) prophylactic mastectomy. I weighed my options. I consulted with a local plastic surgeon who had done breast reconstruction and learned more about what the surgery would entail. After information gathering, I decided to continue surveillance, at least for a few more years until I felt more at ease with my other options.

At 42 I had my second child. I was anxiety ridden during this time about going for so long during the pregnancy and a few months of breastfeeding without doing any breast imaging. My breast cancer risk concerns were always in the back of my mind, but during this time it was particularly worrisome. It was about this time that my husband pointed out an article in *The New York Times* about a woman whom had undergone prophylactic mastectomy and seemed to find some peace with this decision. The breast reconstruction techniques and aesthetic outcomes had made some advances since I had originally done my research several years earlier. At the urging of my husband, who had lost his mother to cancer in her 50s, and now with the recent birth of my daughter and with a ten-year-old son who would be relying on me for many years to come, I decided to give the surgical route another look.

I looked into all the major breast centers around the country and researched the reconstruction techniques. I eventually found a surgical oncologist/plastic surgeon team in Dobbs Ferry, New York, that had a one-step procedure that seemed like it would afford me the breast cancer risk reduction, fast recovery, and the optimal aesthetic results that I wanted. This procedure preserved the skin and nipples, and basically cleaned out the breast tissue, replacing it with an implant. I found out about it on the FORCE website and several former patients generously shared their experiences and post-op photos with me. I read everything I possibly could relating to the procedure and asked countless questions of former patients and the medical providers. I had done all the research I could, explored options, and tried surveillance, and I felt comfortable with going ahead with the prophylactic surgery. I took a deep breath, picked up the phone and scheduled my surgery. In retrospect, this was the single most difficult part of the entire process. In the back of my mind I kept telling myself that I could always cancel the surgery if I changed my mind, but strangely, I felt tremendous relief as soon as the surgery date was set.

I knew that my family would be worried about this decision and was hesitant to discuss my plans very much with them for fear that I might lose my resolve. Some I told before the surgery; some I told months after the surgery was done. Eventually I discussed it with everyone, and though they didn't all agree with me, I felt they were supportive of me. My friends and co-workers were unquestioningly supportive. I explained the surgery plan to my ten-year-old son, discussing what I was going to do and why I was doing it — he listened carefully and then said, "Yep mom, I think you really need to do that surgery and try to get it taken care of." His thoughtful, mature response made me so proud and gave me peace.

In the days leading up to the surgery I was caught up in planning the details — flights, hotels, childcare, work, insurance, pre-op testing, packing, obtaining records — and don't recall allowing myself much time to think about the actual surgery. I knew that this was not a minor surgery and, as with any surgery, there was risk involved for complications, infections, and poor outcome but the risks didn't make me second-guess my decision so I felt that it wasn't worth spending much time thinking about all the problem scenarios. I tried to prepare my husband for the prospect of possible complications, suboptimal outcome, or even the chance of cancer being identified on pathology at the time of surgery. Thankfully none of these things occurred.

Two days before surgery I met with the surgeons, signed consents and had all my final questions answered. The plastic surgeon wanted to get a sense of the reconstructed breast size I wanted to have. I ultimately left it up to him, knowing that with his level of expertise he would know the size that would look pretty and appropriate with my frame size. In retrospect, this was a good decision.

On the day of surgery we woke up early and drove in the cold, dark January morning to the hospital. My husband was calm and positive, as always. I had butterflies and was kind of in a daze but really had no doubts that what I was doing was the right thing. I wasn't even really thinking about it that much, just going through everything moment by moment – registering at the admissions office, meeting with the RN and surgeons, receiving anesthesia, being wheeled into surgery, starting to doze off ... and what seemed like about two minutes later woke up and was told surgery was complete and everything went fine.

I had no pain. My chest was bandaged but normal looking. I was relieved to be done with the surgery and anxious to see my body under the bandages. I had the marcaine ball for pain and some type of IV pain medicine. I was very comfortable. Before long I was able to get out of bed and walk around. The surgeons came in to take off the bandages. I was bruised and misshapen, but I knew it would be months before the implants would settle and soften and take on their final physical appearance. I was hopeful that, though it looked frightening now, it would all look okay someday. Two other post-mastectomy patients strolled down to say hello. I made slow laps around the halls. Aside from some nausea from the pain medication, I felt pretty good. I had a hard time sleeping at night, and took a sleeping pill on my second night, which was a tremendous help. I was released after 2 or 3 days and went to stay at a nearby hotel with my sister, MaryBeth who is also a nurse. My husband and infant daughter returned home to be with my son. Though I felt tired and was a little worried about the nausea returning, the recovery for me was speedy and uneventful.

Feeling well, it was only a day or so after discharge that MaryBeth and I were shopping in the mall, eating lunch at a nearby restaurant, and ... yes, even watching the Super Bowl at a party in the hotel lounge. It all went smoothly, that is, until the Patriots lost .... After a few days I moved out of the hotel and stayed with Amy and her family until my post-op follow up visits were complete and my drains removed; I was cleared to return home when I was about two weeks post-op. The happy hustle of being with Amy and her family was a very pleasant distraction from my recovery process. My pain continued to be very manageable, but I used ibuprofen and narcotic pain medications generously in those first two weeks. I returned to work at my job when I was about three to four weeks post-op. I started with half-days and before long returned full-time to my job.

When back at home I put a futon on the floor so that my infant daughter could crawl over to rest with me – it minimized an lifting

I would need to do to be with her. I still found myself doing too much heavy lifting in those early weeks, but fortunately had no complications.

Over three years have passed now. My recovery progressed normally and I have had no complications. I was fortunate, too, to have a nice aesthetic outcome. I recently saw my pre-op photos and realize how much my appearance has actually improved with the surgery. My post-op breasts are definitely far less sensitive than they were prior to surgery, but I do have some sensitivity and seem to continue to regain it with time.

I don't think about my risk of breast cancer any more. I feel like I've done about all I can do. I know that given the circumstances, I made the right decision for me. I know it isn't the right decision for everyone but I have no regrets and feel fortunate to have had the surgical options and expertise, insurance coverage, support system, and just plain good fortune with how everything turned out for me.

Looking forward, it is my hope that my daughter and nieces won't have to make the same decisions or face these difficult health concerns in their adult lives.

Liz, Age 55

I'm 55 years old. Since my mid-30s I've been plagued with breast cysts, having biopsies done about every 18 to 24 months. Long before I understood the true cancer history in my family, my doctors had told me that I was "high risk" because of my cysts. In the year leading up to my cancer diagnosis I was developing more cysts and developing them at an increasingly faster rate. From March of 2009 to June of 2010, I had eleven biopsies. I felt that my body was announcing its intention to develop cancer and was terrified.

I was pretty sure by February of 2010 that a mastectomy was going to be necessary but the medical people I was dealing with at that point were resistant to discussing it. Because I tested negative for a *BRCA* mutation, even though my mother is *BRCA2+*, the surgeons and genetic counselors I was seeing then patted me on the head and assured me "your risk is the same as the general population."

I knew that could not be true. I was terrified because nobody was giving me any answers about why I was getting so many cysts. I felt doomed to cancer and that nobody was going to help me. I fought hard and moved on to other doctors and kept on until I finally found one, a breast specialist, whom I felt took my concerns seriously. She is the one who found the cancer in June of 2010.

Once the cancer was found my reaction was relief. I remember well when she said "bilateral mastectomy." I was way ahead of her. I wanted an end to what seemed like endless rounds of torture and fear. I'd started hating my breasts, feeling they were the enemy. The cancer was small; it was still early. I was so lucky and I felt that with the surgery I'd be able to finally put it all to rest. When my breast surgeon said "I don't see how we can manage your risk without a bilateral mastectomy," I sat and cried from relief. I told her, "I thought I was going to have to fight you for this . . . ."

In the days leading up to the surgery I was relieved but also felt a lot of anxiety about what kind of pain I'd be facing and what I'd look like afterward. I read a couple of accounts in books written by women who'd had bad experiences and was nauseated at the thought of pain and mutilation. But, at about the time I began to realize that I was probably going to have to face mastectomy, my cousin, who'd had surgery plus reconstruction with implants three years before, emailed me her "before and after" photos.

I was stunned. My cousin's results are fabulous. I pulled those images up and looked at them every time I started to feel nervous — and spent hours on the phone with her and her mother, both cancer survivors, talking about it all. They were both frank in what they said and their assurances that "yes, it's unpleasant but you can get through it" made a lot of difference. They were incredible. They were the glue that kept me from falling apart.

I also spent a lot of time on the FORCE website reading other women's accounts of what they were experiencing. Being able to communicate with other women who were facing the same thing helped immensely; it removed the problem of isolation.

My husband was wonderful. I married a prince. He walked through hell with me. At about the time my cancer was found we learned that his mother was about to die of lung cancer. And at about the time of my mastectomy we learned his stepmother, who he adores, had found breast cancer, too. He was living in "cancer central" for most of 2010. Through it all he showed me in every way possible that I was "priority one." Yes, I married a prince.

I am an American ex-patriot living in Australia. Most of the friends I have here are women I've known three years or less. I did not know what to expect from them, knowing that often people will pull back from a cancer patient because of their own issues and worries. I am still amazed at how quickly my friends encircled me – how they embraced me and supported me through it all. Women I'd known only a few months offered to take me to appointments. They visited, telephoned, brought food and flowers, took me shopping, and just generally showered me with attention and practical assistance.

My friends in the United States were wonderful, too. Although they could not "be here" physically, there were phone calls, emails, and cards. They'd seen me go through many biopsies in the years before coming to Australia. They knew what I'd been through and understood what I was going through. I know a lot of incredible people.

I can't even describe the relief I felt after the surgery. It's like there's been a dark cloud hanging over me for the last twenty years. And now that cloud has lifted. I no longer look into the future and fear it. For the first time I feel truly optimistic and hopeful. I don't have to face having the everlasting crap scared out of me every few months. I'm free of cancer *and* free of the fear. My surgeon tells me my risk of dealing with breast cancer again is something like less than five percent. I'm now way below the risk of the general population.

I'm now six weeks past the exchange surgery, I have cohesive gel implants and nipples reconstructed with skin grafts and although I'm still very uncomfortable at times, I'm thrilled with my result. Having always been a small B cup, I now have D cup breasts — I love my cleavage. My scars are fading beautifully and when I look at myself naked I'm pleased, really pleased. The discomfort is gradually easing and my plastic surgeon assures me that I can expect things to settle down. My breasts are no longer the enemy. I'm starting to love my body again.

In another six weeks I'm going back to the United States for a visit. I've timed the trip so that I can be in my hometown for the annual Susan G. Komen Race for the Cure. I participated in that event in the years before immigrating to Australia. I'll be in it again — this time wearing a pink T-shirt and walking with a group of beautiful women who have supported me long-distance.

Sue, Age 51

I am a previvor. I learned of my *BRCA1+* status after my older sister was diagnosed with breast cancer, elected to be tested, and was found positive. I tested because we lost our oldest sister to breast/ovarian cancer prior to learning the gene was in the family bloodline.

I was determined that prophylactic mastectomy was the right thing for me to do. So, the wait was awful ... I just wanted to be done with the surgery and get on with living. I was worried I would get cancer before the surgery would reduce my risk. I felt awful to be mutilating my healthy body. I am an active person who has strived to take good care of myself. I was in the best physical shape of my life having lost a fair amount of weight during the prior year and had gotten into an exercise routine that had me healthy and in top fighting form. I thought I was doing it to look good; I didn't realize I was preparing for a larger event. Anyway, I was always prideful of my appearance, and knew I would not be the same after — even with the best of outcomes. I talked to my husband and was *very* fortunate that he was supportive of my decision, and willing to talk about his own emotions regarding the upcoming changes. It helped so much to have him understanding of the need, yet willing to grieve the loss that was also coming, and be willing to talk to me about both notions.

Emotionally, I kept remembering my oldest sister, and all she went through with her cancers and her ultimate death, and my surviving sister going through chemo. In my mind I knew I had to act *now* to honor them. I feel their diagnosis/treatments were a gift to me, grabbing my attention, getting me to do something, enabling me to act proactively rather than having to react to a diagnosis as they did. How could I *not* take what they taught me and use it to save myself the pain? I knew deeply I was doing the right thing ... I just had to get through it.

So, my surgery was scheduled for two days after a wonderful family vacation with my hubby and children. That kept my mind off it beautifully. When we returned, I was too busy getting last minute things done: kids back to college, pre-op appointments, unpacking from the trip, packing for the hospital, organizing the house, helping my boss be ready for my absence. I didn't have time to dwell on it *until* the morning of surgery. I was a basket case until they put the medicine into the IV to help me relax – then I fell asleep. My next memory was waking up after it was all over. I was instantly, totally at peace.

My friends and family were very supportive of my decision, and in "awe of my courage" was what I often heard. Also, I would say that anyone who was not supportive had the common courtesy of keeping their thoughts to themselves. I say this because there were friends/relatives I expected to hear from after my information hit the streets who were silent, and remain so.

I get frustrated some days – it has only been twelve weeks as of today – because I am not physically back to my pre-surgery fitness level. But I am confident this will come. I am pleased with my appearance, I look like my pre-surgery self in clothes. Naked ... I sigh ... I had beautiful unblemished breasts before this; they are a bit scary now. But my husband is comfortable with them, and my attitude improves each day as the scars fade.

Laurie, Age 39

I am 4.5 weeks post-mastectomy and just started the expansion/ reconstruction process. I am a previvor and this was a prophylactic procedure. My family is spread across the United Kingdom and Ireland and I did not grow up with any awareness of a familial risk or prevalence of cancer. I got to know this side of the family in the last three years and along with that came my knowledge of the *BRCA1* mutation in the family. I was tested last year at age 38. I leaned toward surgery from the first but did spend six months reading, meeting with doctors, talking to other women, and reviewing the FORCE website. My friends and family had mixed responses. Many people were loathe to acknowledge the severity of the situation and characterized my decision for surgery as extreme or an over-reaction. I quickly stopped discussing the situation with these people, my own father included who carried the mutation. I've reached the conclusion that people tend to react based on their own personality types and fears. I've always been a do-er and it was inconceivable to me to merely sit back and wait to get cancer. My husband was very supportive of surgery from the beginning.

In the days leading up to the surgery, I felt as though it was all a bit unreal. It was difficult to truly process the concept of operating on a healthy body emotionally. I relied heavily on my intellect to get me through and tried to be kind to myself when I had moments of anxiety and anger. I sought the support of a psychologist, talked to women who had been through this, and read the FORCE message boards regularly. As the surgery date neared, I read the FORCE website daily and generally spent time with my husband, distancing myself a bit from anyone who may not have understood my choice. My sister tested positive a few months after I did and although she has yet to make a decision about her own course of action, she and I did talk a lot about my decision. We tiptoed around it at first as she was extremely resistant to the idea of surgery. She is heavily in favor of alternative medicine but we were ultimately able to find common ground after she met with an oncologist. She went in expecting to find a middle ground between surgery and surveillance and was shocked to discover that such a middle ground does not exist. She apologized to me for ever making me feel judged for choosing surgery and we've talked a lot more about the situation since then.

The surgery is still very close, so I'm not sure that I have made it through the emotional process that this surgery entails, but here goes: The first two weeks after the surgery I felt really good. I was medicated for the pain and able to start walking almost immediately. About three weeks after the surgery I got an infection in my right breast. The surgeon wanted to operate a second time and remove the expander, thereby waiting six months to reconstruct that side. I did not see it coming and was absolutely devastated at the idea of being without a breast for so long. More than that, the idea of another surgery seemed unthinkable. I cried in the hallway of the doctor's office while my husband tried to hold me (gently — you can't hug after a mastectomy very well). I felt ridiculous for being so upset because women who have had breast cancer deal with far worse than what I was facing but I was truly devastated at the idea of going back under anesthesia, going back to the hospital, and experiencing more pain. Fortunately, I was able to avoid that surgery and have recovered from the infection almost completely. I am now starting the expansion process; I had my first fill yesterday. I have started to get some energy back; I'm allowed to walk a mile a day. During the days when I thought I was headed back to the hospital, the weight of the surgery really seemed to hit me emotionally. I would be up all night thinking and once at 2 A.M., I started to cry as I thought about the fact that I would never be the same. I have never been a woman who identified much with my breasts in terms of body image — they were not very large and as a result I think I didn't pay much attention them. And yet, I felt sadness for the first time that night thinking about the times I had been touched and appreciated the breasts that were now gone. And here I sit, a week past that moment and I realize that I have finally begun the emotional process of accepting the choice I made. I have no regrets, but do allow myself moments of sadness.

On being a previvor, I'm glad someone came up with a word because throughout this process I have felt that many of my reactions are petty and unimportant compared to the women in my family and the women I have met who have survived breast cancer. However, my reactions of anger, sadness, and frustration have been very real. Basically, I put this decision in the category of real adult choices in my life that is mine and mine alone. I chose to remove my breasts, I chose to minimize my risk of getting breast cancer, and I choose to live as long a life as I can. It all comes back to that for me. Once I'm through this, I will turn to the ovarian cancer risk. I know that I will ultimately have to remove my ovaries, but that's for next year. This year, I get new breasts for my fortieth birthday.

Carey

In January of 2006 I heard that my father's first cousins in the United Kingdom had been part of a study at Oxford that found a new *BRCA* mutation in our family. I started looking into being tested. A month later, I went to my gynecologist thinking I had a urinary tract infection but, long story short, I was on the table by March 31 having debulking surgery for Stage 3C ovarian cancer. We proceeded under the assumption that I was *BRCA+* until I was tested and we knew for certain. I finished chemotherapy and started looking into having a prophylactic bilateral mastectomy. My gynecologic-oncologist/surgeon cleared me for surgery. I went to see "the" breast surgeon at the same place where I had had my ovarian cancer surgery. I knew I wanted DIEP flap reconstruction. But the surgeon refused to perform the mastectomy, saying that I was at greater risk of an ovarian cancer recurrence than developing a new primary and "you'll be under such strict surveillance that we'd discover anything before it was mortal." It was the surveillance that had convinced me that I wanted a prophylactic bilateral mastectomy in the first place — mammograms, more images, ultrasound, biopsy, wait for results ... it was taking years off my life. (In retrospect) I really don't think the breast surgeon thought I'd survive long enough to make it worth it.

It was spring of 2007 when I got in to see a new surgeon and got things set up. We planned to do the surgery in October of 2007 because everyone was convinced there was no reason to hurry. But in September of 2007 they found an ovarian cancer recurrence. I went on trial with Avastin so I couldn't have the prophylactic mastectomy surgery. But part of the Avastin trial involved having a CT scan that ended up showing a mass in my breast: Stage 2B breast cancer. It was discovered four months after the last mammogram/ultrasound and two months from the next scheduled breast MRI. I had to get out of the Avastin study, have the mastectomy, and then go back to regular chemotherapy for the ovarian cancer.

I did have the DIEP flap and have been pleased. But now, almost three years later, I am still angry that I didn't manage to have a completely prophylactic mastectomy. I had cancerous lymph nodes removed so I am at risk for lymphedema and I can't use my right arm for needlesticks, etc.

I founded Teal Toes (www.tealtoes.org) to raise awareness of ovarian cancer. Teal is the color for ovarian cancer, and I discovered that painting toe nails teal tends to spark conversation that allows for ovarian cancer facts to be conveyed. I send out wallet-sized cards with the ovarian cancer symptoms to anyone who asks. I'm pretty sure that I have ordered close to 100,000 cards in the last three years.

I am constantly shocked at the lack of knowledge regarding the *BRCA* link with ovarian cancer. I meet young women who know that they are at risk due to family history for breast cancer but have no idea about ovarian cancer. I also think that it is important for people to be aware that it is possible that new mutations have been discovered since they were tested — or will be discovered.

E.

I am a previvor. I was 39 when I got my positive genetic test results back, married, with two kids. When I walked into the room to hear my test results, I knew that if they were positive I would have a prophylactic bilateral mastectomy. It was a no brainer for me, as my sense of self and feelings of womanhood were not tied up with having breasts. While the decision to have the surgery was an easy one for me to make, anticipating the actual surgery, the recovery, and the impact on my family — especially my kids — made me apprehensive. I had never had major surgery before, and my kids had never been away from both parents at the same time.

I got my test results at the end of April and, being the practical-minded person I am, I decided I wanted to have the mastectomy surgery over with and me healed enough to take care of my kids by the time they were out of school for the summer. That required pretty quick action on my part, and some luck with scheduling of doctors and the operating room. From the time I got my test results back to the time I was wheeled into the operating room was twelve days. I spent those twelve days finding both a breast surgeon and a plastic surgeon I trusted and deciding on if I even wanted reconstruction and if so, what type. I live in an area with many fine doctors, so finding a team I trusted was easy. I decided on having expanders placed at the time of my mastectomy, with an eventual trade-out to gummy bear silicone implants. At the time I had my mastectomy this was the least invasive breast reconstruction option in my area with the quickest healing time. And as I wasn't entirely sure I really wanted/needed reconstruction, I felt it would be easy for me to change my mind and have the implants removed at a future date if I desired.

In the days leading up to my mastectomy I was more worried about organizing the logistics for my kids and husband, and figuring out where my kids would be while my husband and I were at the hospital overnight. The kids were five and seven at the time, so still fairly young. I think because I was so busy getting everything all straightened out for them, I didn't spend much time thinking about me. This was probably some sort of coping mechanism on my part. But I never wavered in my decision and the thought never crossed my mind to back out of it or to wait a little longer.

I also needed to talk with my kids about what was happening, and why. Not only would I be gone and their routine disrupted, but when I was back home I would be taking heavy-duty pain medications and not acting like the mommy they were used to. I am a medical professional, and strongly feel that telling my kids the truth, in an age-appropriate manner, is the best way to deal with medical situations. At the time I was planning my mastectomy, my mother was undergoing chemotherapy for breast cancer, and my mother was very open with the kids about letting them touch her bald head and talking about the medicine that made her feel bad but was helping to kill the cancer in her body. My kids were, therefore, familiar with the word cancer, and with cancer treatments. My husband and I decided that we would talk with the kids about how I have a genetic mutation, like a bad bug, that could give me cancer like grandma, and we didn't want that to happen, so I would be getting a surgery to take my breasts off and replace them with something like water balloons on the inside. We also talked with them about how I would be taking some medicine so that I wouldn't feel much pain while my body was healing, but the medicine would make me sleepy and act a bit funny for a little bit of time. And we talked about how they were having a special treat — sleepovers at a friend's house – while Mommy was in the hospital. We answered the questions they had, and left it at that.

My family and friends were very supportive. With my mom's recent cancer diagnosis, her second, my family and husband all felt it was the right decision. My friends, and the teachers and parents at my kids' schools were incredible! I was very open with everyone about what was happening and why, and if anyone disagreed with me, they didn't tell me personally.

After my surgery I was caught off guard by how much I mourned the loss of my breasts because they were what had nourished my children. Both of my kids breastfed for years and years, and I have very strong positive memories of that time in our lives. Losing my breasts meant losing that physical part of my memories. Now, my new body is just my body. This is how it looks. I have horizontal scars across each breast and haven't had nipple reconstruction, and that is just how they are. My kids have no memory of me looking any different than how I look now. We still, as a family, talk about me having the *BRCA* mutation. We talk in a casual way about it, wanting to keep the subject alive in the minds of our kids, as someday they will have to decide if they will get tested. My husband and I hope that my example of normalizing the surgeries and living a healthy life after the surgeries (I've also had my ovaries out) will help our kids deal with the potential of having a *BRCA* mutation themselves in a positive, proactive manner and not from a position of fear. My body now is the new normal for everyone in my family. No regrets. Ever. At all.

Gillian

In May of 2006 I made a choice for my future. Three years earlier, I had been diagnosed with the genetic mutation known as *BRCA2*, putting me at a much higher risk of breast and ovarian cancer than the general population. At that time I chose to have surgery known as bilateral salpingo-oophorectomy (BSO) with a hysterectomy to reduce my risk of breast and ovarian cancer. After having yearly surveillance since I was 30 years old, I decided to have a bilateral prophylactic mastectomy (BPM). At the same time, our family decided to knock down and rebuild our old home. Similarities between the circumstances were not lost on us! I was surgically removing as much breast tissue as possible and unlike our home, I decided on no reconstruction.

My decision was based on many things including length of surgery, recovery time, and the need for future surgeries. My own goal for the surgery was simply to reduce my risk of cancer being found in my breasts or ovaries. I had no ovaries but my breasts still reminded me of the time bomb that had claimed my mother when she was 43 years young and I was only twelve. Her mother had died early, as had her mother, now I was empowered to stay as well as I could thanks to the latest medical research.

With this knowledge of the gene mutation I received help, both medical and psychological, from specialist doctors, family and friends, my faith, and on-line at Facing Our Risk Of Cancer (FORCE). I chose to surround myself with encouraging people, wrote in my journal, went on holidays, wrote lists, and read other women's stories, trials, and hopes, as well as listening to my own voice.

My children, when I had the first surgery in 2003, were 18 and 14 years old, so when the next surgery occurred, they saw it as a time when I was doing whatever it took to be around for them. I was doing the best I could and they were seeing a new home emerge on the same block of land they already loved. My children gave me the enthusiasm and energy to continue while my husband always continued to care and reassure me that I was doing the best [thing] not only for me but for him, too. They are my best incentive and my greatest supporters.

To prepare for each of the surgeries I kept the facts before me and reminded myself of strategies I used personally to cope, from when I was just twelve when my mother died. Some needed refining, some I needed to throw away, but I have learned more about myself through this time than I could have ever imagined. I was in the fortunate situation of being able to choose doctors, specialists, and hospitals that all understood and encouraged me about the available medical options. Rather than waiting for a cancer diagnosis, I was now empowered to take steps to undertake preventive surgery. I took care of the family time bomb while I was healthy and my family was in a good place – well, a few, in reality!

In the days leading up to BPM day, as we called it, I wrote letters to my children, tidied the home as though I wasn't about to knock it down, and organized things for when I was recovering. I wrote questions for my doctors and nurses and talked to many close friends. The others on FORCE really understood where I was and how to give me what I needed without judgment or even need of thanks. It was the community that got me where I was and accepted me and wanted the best for me, just because they were also facing these moments. It was a rollercoaster of emotions that was hard to describe to others, but those on FORCE also knew of the "ride" and helped me see the big picture.

My body is not what it was, neither is my home. Both are much better and ready to cope with more of life's adventures. Plastic surgery was not for me and I am more than happy with wearing prostheses when I want to and swimming with none. I have recognized the importance of really watching my body for signs of wear and tear, and nurturing it so that I can live well. Physically I am different but my mother would have been so happy to have my options. Not everything went according to my plan; I actually had two surgeries to remove breast tissue, an infection and slow healing of my incisions, and we moved three times in a year before our new home was complete.

I recently had the privilege of watching my beautiful daughter marry a wonderful man. I was the first mother in four generations of my immediate family to be able to see her daughter marry. My daughter does not carry the *BRCA2* gene and her future is already looking brighter with her mother being here to cheer her on from the sidelines. My son at 21 is still to test and that will be a whole new chapter of our story.

So the choice of a BPM was one I've been glad to be able to make, pleased I had options, and confident my own voice has been heard. I made decisions that I may not have made at a different time, but today as I write this I am happy with my health and the way I have been able to reduce my risk of breast and ovarian cancer. Knowing about my genetic mutation has actually presented me with a future and for that I will always be grateful.

5

Post-Surgical
Instructions

Post-Operative Instructions and Precautions

Patient Name: _____

Physician: _____

Physician Telephone: _____

Medications: _____

Limitations in Arm Movements:

_____

_____

Other Activity Restrictions:

_____

_____

Do not lift anything over _____ lbs.

Wound Care Instructions:

_____

_____

Empty drains _____ times per day.

Showering: **IS / IS NOT** permitted. (*Circle one*)

Do not drive for _____ weeks or until drains are removed.

Notes: _____

_____

**Recommended follow-up appointment in _____ days. Call
your physician to schedule this upon discharge.**

Drainage Chart

Use this chart to record drainage amounts daily. Be sure to label your drains 1, 2, 3, and 4 with a permanent marker. This will help you keep track of how much fluid is draining from each drain. Bring this information with you to your post-operative visits.

DATE / TIME	DRAIN 1	DRAIN 2	DRAIN 3	DRAIN 4
A.M.				
P.M. – 1				
P.M. – 2				
Total Day 1				
A.M.				
P.M. – 1				
P.M. – 2				
Total Day 2				
A.M.				
P.M. – 1				
P.M. – 2				
Total Day 3				

DATE / TIME	DRAIN 1	DRAIN 2	DRAIN 3	DRAIN 4
A.M.				
P.M. – 1				
P.M. – 2				
Total Day 4				
A.M.				
P.M. – 1				
P.M. – 2				
Total Day 5				
A.M.				
P.M. – 1				
P.M. – 2				
Total Day 6				
A.M.				
P.M. – 1				
P.M. – 2				
Total Day 7				

DATE / TIME	DRAIN 1	DRAIN 2	DRAIN 3	DRAIN 4
A.M.				
P.M. – 1				
P.M. – 2				
Total Day 8				
A.M.				
P.M. – 1				
P.M. – 2				
Total Day 9				
A.M.				
P.M. – 1				
P.M. – 2				
Total Day 10				
A.M.				
P.M. – 1				
P.M. – 2				
Total Day 11				

DATE / TIME	DRAIN 1	DRAIN 2	DRAIN 3	DRAIN 4
A.M.				
P.M. – 1				
P.M. – 2				
Total Day 12				
A.M.				
P.M. – 1				
P.M. – 2				
Total Day 13				
A.M.				
P.M. – 1				
P.M. – 2				
Total Day 14				
A.M.				
P.M. – 1				
P.M. – 2				
Total Day 15				

DATE / TIME	DRAIN 1	DRAIN 2	DRAIN 3	DRAIN 4
A.M.				
P.M. – 1				
P.M. – 2				
Total Day 16				
A.M.				
P.M. – 1				
P.M. – 2				
Total Day 17				
A.M.				
P.M. – 1				
P.M. – 2				
Total Day 18				
A.M.				
P.M. – 1				
P.M. – 2				
Total Day 19				

DATE / TIME	DRAIN 1	DRAIN 2	DRAIN 3	DRAIN 4
A.M.				
P.M. – 1				
P.M. – 2				
Total Day 20				
A.M.				
P.M. – 1				
P.M. – 2				
Total Day 21				

Medication/Activity Log

Use this chart to keep track of when you take medications and empty your drains. Record anything else that you think may be important throughout the day and bring this with you when you follow up with your physician.

TIME	SAMPLE 1	DAY 1
MIDNIGHT – 4 A.M.		
4 A.M. – 8 A.M.	Percocet – 4 A.M. Cipro – 7 A.M. Drains emptied 7:00 A.M.	
8 A.M. – NOON	Percocet – 10 A.M.	
NOON – 4 P.M.	Drains emptied 2:00 P.M. Percocet 2:45 P.M.	
4 P.M. – 8 P.M.		
8 P.M. – MIDNIGHT	Cipro – 7 P.M. Drains emptied 10:00 P.M. Percocet 8:30 P.M. Ambien 11 P.M.	

TIME	DAY 2	DAY 3
MIDNIGHT – 4 A.M.		
4 A.M. – 8 A.M.		
8 A.M. – NOON		
NOON – 4 P.M.		
4 P.M. – 8 P.M.		
8 P.M. – MIDNIGHT		

TIME	DAY 4	DAY 5
MIDNIGHT – 4 A.M.		
4 A.M. – 8 A.M.		
8 A.M. – NOON		
NOON – 4 P.M.		
4 P.M. – 8 P.M.		
8 P.M. – MIDNIGHT		

TIME	DAY 6	DAY 7
MIDNIGHT – 4 A.M.		
4 A.M. – 8 A.M.		
8 A.M. – NOON		
NOON – 4 P.M.		
4 P.M. – 8 P.M.		
8 P.M. – MIDNIGHT		

TIME	DAY 8	DAY 9
MIDNIGHT – 4 A.M.		
4 A.M. – 8 A.M.		
8 A.M. – NOON		
NOON – 4 P.M.		
4 P.M. – 8 P.M.		
8 P.M. – MIDNIGHT		

TIME	DAY 10	DAY 11
MIDNIGHT – 4 A.M.		
4 A.M. – 8 A.M.		
8 A.M. – NOON		
NOON – 4 P.M.		
4 P.M. – 8 P.M.		
8 P.M. – MIDNIGHT		

TIME	DAY 12	DAY 13
MIDNIGHT – 4 A.M.		
4 A.M. – 8 A.M.		
8 A.M. – NOON		
NOON – 4 P.M.		
4 P.M. – 8 P.M.		
8 P.M. – MIDNIGHT		

TIME	DAY 14	DAY 15
MIDNIGHT – 4 A.M.		
4 A.M. – 8 A.M.		
8 A.M. – NOON		
NOON – 4 P.M.		
4 P.M. – 8 P.M.		
8 P.M. – MIDNIGHT		

TIME	DAY 16	DAY 17
MIDNIGHT – 4 A.M.		
4 A.M. – 8 A.M.		
8 A.M. – NOON		
NOON – 4 P.M.		
4 P.M. – 8 P.M.		
8 P.M. – MIDNIGHT		

TIME	DAY 18	DAY 19
MIDNIGHT – 4 A.M.		
4 A.M. – 8 A.M.		
8 A.M. – NOON		
NOON – 4 P.M.		
4 P.M. – 8 P.M.		
8 P.M. – MIDNIGHT		

TIME	DAY 20	DAY 21
MIDNIGHT – 4 A.M.		
4 A.M. – 8 A.M.		
8 A.M. – NOON		
NOON – 4 P.M.		
4 P.M. – 8 P.M.		
8 P.M. – MIDNIGHT		

Post-Operative Outpatient Visit Number 1

Date/Time: _____

Physician: _____

Address: _____

Questions/Concerns Since Last Visit: _____
_____
_____

Any Changes in Precautions/Restrictions?: _____
_____
_____

Medication Changes: _____
_____
_____

Wound Care Instructions: _____
_____

Range of Motion Exercises: _____
_____

Other: _____

Next follow-up visit in _____ (days) with_____.

Notes

Post-Operative Outpatient Visit Number 2

Date/Time: _____

Physician: _____

Address: _____

Questions/Concerns Since Last Visit: _____

_____

_____

Any Changes in Precautions/Restrictions?: _____

_____

_____

Medication Changes: _____

_____

_____

Wound Care Instructions: _____

_____

Range of Motion Exercises: _____

_____

Other: _____

Next follow-up visit in _____ (days) with_____.

Notes

Post-Operative Outpatient Visit Number 3

Date/Time: _____

Physician: _____

Address: _____

Questions/Concerns Since Last Visit: _____

_____

_____

Any Changes in Precautions/Restrictions?: _____

_____

_____

Medication Changes: _____

_____

_____

Wound Care Instructions: _____

_____

Range of Motion Exercises: _____

_____

Other: _____

Next follow-up visit in _____ (days) with_____.

Notes

Post-Operative Outpatient Visit Number 4

Date/Time: _____

Physician: _____

Address: _____

Questions/Concerns Since Last Visit: _____

_____

_____

Any Changes in Precautions/Restrictions?: _____

_____

_____

Medication Changes: _____

_____

_____

Wound Care Instructions: _____

_____

Range of Motion Exercises: _____

_____

Other: _____

Next follow-up visit in _____ (days) with_____.

Notes

Glossary of Terms

Adhesive Capsulitis. Also called frozen shoulder syndrome, a loss of range of motion due to inflammation of the capsule of the shoulder joint.

Adjuvant Chemotherapy. Chemotherapy that is given after tumor removal to help ensure that any microscopic cancer cells have been destroyed.

Alveoli. Air sacs in the lungs.

Ankle Pumps. An exercise done after surgery to help reduce the risk of blood clots.

Atypical Ductal Hyperplasia. An abnormal, but not cancerous, overgrowth of cells in the milk ducts.

Autologous Reconstruction. A type of breast reconstruction that involves the use of the patient's own tissue.

Axillary Lymph Nodes. Lymph nodes located in the underarm area. Axillary lymph node dissection is when some or all lymph nodes in this area are removed.

Axillary Lymph Node Dissection. When lymph nodes are removed from the axilla (the underarm area).

Axillary Web Syndrome. A webbing or cording that sometimes develops in the axilla and along the length of the arm after lymph node injury.

Baker Grading System. Classification criteria used to determine the extent of capsular contracture.

Bed Mobility. Techniques for moving easily and safely in and out of bed.

Bilateral Mastectomy. Removal of breast tissue on both breasts.

Biopsy. A type of procedure that removes a small amount of tissue to test it for cancer.

BI-RADS. The Breast Imaging Reporting and Data System is a system radiologists use to classify mammogram results.

BRCA1 and BRCA2. Breast cancer susceptibility gene 1 and breast cancer susceptibility gene 2. Individuals who test "positive" for *BRCA1* or *2* have increased risk for breast and ovarian cancer.

Breast Conserving Surgery. Surgery that saves as much healthy breast tissue as possible. A lumpectomy is considered breast conserving surgery.

Breast Form. A breast prosthesis that may be used after mastectomy. Usually made of silicone, foam, or fiberfill depending on a woman's stage of recovery after mastectomy.

Breast Implant. A prosthesis that is implanted under skin and muscle to form a breast mound after mastectomy.

Capsular Contracture. Tightening of the scar tissue surounding a breast implant that may lead to deformity.

Capsulectomy. Surgery to remove scar tissue surrounding a breast implant when capsular contracture has developed.

Certified Fitter-Mastectomy (CF-m). A certified professional who is specially trained in fitting breast prostheses after mastectomy.

Chemotherapy. A type of cancer treatment that uses drugs to destroy or slow the growth of cancer cells.

Cohesive Gel Implants. Also known as "gummy bear" implants, these implants are made up of soft, solid silicone gel material throughout.

Dangle. Sitting up at the edge of the bed for a few minutes in order to let your blood pressure adjust to the change in position after surgery or immobility.

DCIS. *See* Ductal Carcinoma in Situ.

Debridement. The process of removing dead tissue around a wound.

Deep Inferior Epigrastric Perforator Flap (DIEP). A flap surgery that moves tissue, fat, small blood vessels, and skin from the abdomen and relocates it to the chest to form the breast mound.

Direct to Implant Reconstruction. A type of breast reconstruction that involves placing implants immediately after the mastectomy is performed.

Donor Site. In autologous or "flap" breast reconstruction procedures, the donor site is the area from which the tissue that will ultimately become the breast mound is taken.

Doppler Ultrasound. A type of ultrasound that can be used both pre- and post-operatively to assess tissue blood flow for flap procedures.

Drain(s). Tubes inserted during mastectomy that drain excess blood and fluids. Jackson-Pratt type drains are most often used during mastectomy.

Drain Management. The process of caring for and emptying the drains.

Dressing Stick. An assistive device that can be used to help with dressing, particularly when a patient has difficulty reaching or bending down.

Ductal Carcinoma in Situ (DCIS). When cancerous cells are located within the milk ducts of the breast and have not invaded the surrounding breast tissue.

Durable Medical Equipment. Medical equipment such as hospital beds, shower and bath chairs that can be used repeatedly.

Energy Conservation Principles. Common sense principles for conserving the energy we use throughout the day during basic self-care, home management, and work tasks.

Fill. The process of injecting saline into the valve on a tissue expander in order to increase the size of the reconstructed breast.

Flap Procedure. A procedure for breast reconstruction that involves use of the patient's own tissue.

Free TRAM Flap. A type of transverse rectus abdominus flap (TRAM). With this procedure an area of tissue is removed from the rectus abdominus muscle and reattached at the reconstruction site.

Frozen Shoulder Syndrome. *See* Adhesive Capsulitis.

Genetic Counselor. A person who is trained in genetics and counsels families and individuals about hereditary diseases and syndromes.

Guarding. The tendency to be over-protective of a limb after injury or surgery. Guarding can contribute to development of lymphedema and decreased range of motion.

Hematoma. A localized mass of blood under tissue.

Incentive Spirometer. A device that measures lung capacity. Used after surgeries to keep lungs clear and promote deep breathing.

Intermittent Pneumatic Compression Boots. Devices worn on the calves that help maintain circulation to reduce the postsurgical risk of blood clot.

Intubation. A tube that is placed in the patient's airway during surgery to assist with breathing.

Invasive Ductal Carcinoma. Also called invasive ductal cancer. With this type of breast cancer, the cancer has spread beyond the milk ducts and has invaded the surrounding tissue.

Jackson-Pratt Drains™. A device most commonly used after mastectomy to drain excess blood and fluid from the incision sites.

Latissimus Dorsi Flap. A type of flap procedure that reroutes the latissimus dorsi muscle of the back to form the breast mound.

Lipofilling. The process of liposuctioning fat from one area of the body and then injecting into the reconstructed breast in order to improve contour and cosmetic outcome.

Lobules. Small areas within the breast tissue where milk is made.

Local Anesthesia. A medication for pain control that is used in a specific area of the body.

Lock Out Interval. When using a patient-controlled analgesic pump, it is the maximum number of doses a person can give him-/herself within a specific time period.

Long-Handled Shoe Horn. A shoe horn with an extended handle that can be used when a patient has difficulty reaching his or her feet.

Lumpectomy. A surgical procedure when only the cancerous tumor and a small amount of normal surrounding tissue is removed from the breast. The nipple and areolar complex is typically not removed with this type of surgery.

Lymphedema. A swelling that can occur in the chest or arm when the flow of the lymphatic system is impaired. This may be due to lymph node removal or injury.

Lymphoscintigraphy. *See* Sentinel Lymph Node Mapping.

Lymph Node. A tiny, bean like structure that is part of the lymphatic system. Lymph nodes pick up and move lymph fluid through our bodies.

Marcaine Ball. A device that delivers local anesthetic directly into the breast area over a period of two to three days.

Margin. The areas of healthy tissue surrounding a cancerous tumor.

Mastectomy Bra. A bra that is designed specifically for post-mastectomy use and may include a pocket for holding a breast form.

Medical Oncologist. A physician who specializes in treating cancer.

Microsurgery. The process of reattaching tissues including small structures such as blood vessels using a microscope.

Modified Radical Mastectomy. With this type of mastectomy the breast tissue, nipple areolar complex, and the lower axillary lymph nodes are removed.

Neuropathic Pain. Chronic pain that is the result of damage to nerves.

Nipple Areolar Complex (NAC). The area of the breast that includes both the nipple and the areola.

Nipple Reconstruction. A surgical procedure that involves recreating a nipple from the patient's own tissue.

Nipple Sparing Mastectomy. A type of mastectomy that removes the underlying tissue but preserves the nipple areolar complex.

Occupational Therapist. A health care professional who helps patients to achieve their maximum level of independence in the face of a variety of disabilities and post-surgical conditions.

One Step Surgery. Also known as direct to implant reconstruction.

Orthostatic Hypotension. When blood pressure falls rapidly due to rapid change in position. May cause dizziness and lightheadedness.

Pathology. The study of disease processes within tissue.

Patient Controlled Analgesic (PCA) Pump. The patient controls an IV pump that delivers pain medication.

Pectoralis Muscles. Refers to two muscles located on the chest, the smaller underlying muscle is the pectoralis minor; the larger, outermost muscle is the pectoralis major.

Pedicle TRAM Flap. A type of flap procedure whereby the transverse rectus abdominus muscle (TRAM) is rerouted up under the skin to form a breast mound.

Peripheral Neuropathy. Damage to nerves of the peripheral nervous system. Peripheral nerves supply our bodies with sensation.

Phantom Sensation. When a person continues to feel sensation in a body part that has been removed such as a breast.

Plastic Surgeon. A physician who specializes in cosmetic and reconstructive surgeries. This type of physician may specialize in performing breast reconstruction surgery.

Post-Operative. The period after surgery.

Previvor. An individual who is at risk for developing cancer due to a hereditary condition such as *BRCA1* or *2*.

Precautions. The rules, limitations, and restrictions that physicians give their patients based on the patient's illness or post-surgical condition.

Prophylactic Mastectomy. When a mastectomy is performed prior to a breast cancer diagnosis. Prophylactic mastectomy is often undertaken as a risk-reducing procedure when there is a strong hereditary link with breast cancer.

Prosthesis. A breast form that can be worn after mastectomy to give an appearance of a breast as well as to provide balance and symmetry.

Protective Posturing. *See* Guarding.

Ptosis. Sagging of the breasts.

Radiation Therapy. The use of radiation to kill cancer cells.

Radical Mastectomy. Removal of the skin, breast tissue, nipple, some or all of the underlying chest muscle, and all of the axillary lymph nodes.

Reacher. An assistive device used for reaching far away objects. Often used when a patient has limited range of motion.

Re-excision. Also called "clearing the margins," re-excision is when a patient undergoes a second surgery to ensure that all cancerous tissue has been removed and suitable healthy margins have been established.

Regeneration of Nerves. The process of regrowth and repair of nerves.

Sanguineous Fluid. Blood.

Scar Massage. The process of massaging newly formed scar tissue to create a smooth appearance and prevent adhesions.

Scoliosis. Curvature of the spine.

Serosanguineous Fluid. Blood and serous fluid.

SGAP. *See* Superior Gluteal Artery Flap.

Sentinel Lymph Node. The first lymph node(s) that drains lymph away from the breast.

Sentinel Lymph Node Biopsy. When the sentinel lymph node is removed and biopsied to determine if cancer has progressed to the lymph nodes.

Sentinel Lymph Node Mapping. A radiological procedure using a radioisotope and/or blue dye; often performed in conjunction with mastectomy to identify the sentinel lymph node(s) for the purposes of biopsy.

Serous Fluid. A transparent, watery fluid.

Skin Sparing Mastectomy. A type of mastectomy that removes the underlying breast tissue and the nipple and areola but conserves the overlying skin to the greatest extent possible.

Simple Mastectomy. A type of mastectomy that removes underlying breast tissue and the nipple areolar complex.

Sock Aid. An assistive device that patients can use to help them put on socks when they have difficulty reaching their feet.

Staging of Cancer. Describes the extent of a cancer in an individual's body.

Steri-strips™. Strips of tape that are often used as an alternative to stitches. Steri-strips usually fall off on their own within ten days.

Superior Gluteal Artery Perforator Flap. Transplants a portion of the gluteal muscles of the buttocks to form the breast mound.

Surgical Oncologist. A surgeon who specializes in removing cancerous tissue.

Surveillance. Screening and testing to detect cancer in its earliest stages when it is most treatable.

Symmastia. Breast implants that are positioned too close together.

Tamoxifen. An oral medication that interferes with estrogen production. Often used in pre-menopausal women with early stage breast cancer.

Tissue Expander. A small, balloon-like sac that is placed behind the chest muscle during surgery and gradually, over a period of months, filled with saline to achieve the desired breast size.

Tissue Matrix. A type of tissue that can be used to increase area of coverage with breast implants. This tissue acts like a scaffolding upon which the patient's own tissues grow.

Transverse Rectus Abominus (TRAM) Flap. A type of flap procedure that uses the rectus abdominus muscle of the abdomen to create the breast mound in reconstruction.

Urinary Catheter. A thin tube inserted into a patient's bladder to drain urine.

Visual Analog Pain Scale. A tool used to rate a patient's pain level. The patient is asked to place their pain on a continuum ranging from 0 to 10, with 0 being no pain and 10 being the most extreme pain.

The Women's Health and Cancer Rights Act (WHCRA) of 1998. WHCRA is legislation that requires health insurance companies that cover mastectomy to also offer coverage for breast reconstruction and certain post-operative complications.

Products We Love

Best Friends For Life (www.bfflco.com/). Designed to improve the patient experience, the BFFL bag includes all of the post-mastectomy supplies you will need during your recovery including the Axilla Pilla™, drain supplies, toiletries, scar cream, and more.

Leachco Back-N-Belly Pillow (www.leachco.com/). Mastectomy patients swear by this pillow for a good night's sleep at home after surgery.

Rub-On Nipples (www.Rub-on Nipples.com). Three-dimensional temporary nipple and areola tattoos that come in a variety of colors. They are easy to apply and a great option if you have had reconstructive surgery but have chosen not to have nipple tattoos or are between surgeries.

Endnotes

1. Susan M. Love, M.D., and Karen Lindsey, *Dr. Susan Love's Breast Book*, *4th ed.*, Cambridge, MA: Da Capo Press, 2005, p. 103.
2. American Cancer Society, "Surgery for Breast Cancer," (http://www.cancer.org/Cancer/BreastCancer/OverviewGuide/breast-cancer-overview-treating-surgery) accessed June 2011.
3. *Stedman's Medical Dictionary*. 2006. 28th ed., Baltimore, MD: Lippincott, Williams & Wilkins, p. 1160.
4. *Stedman's*, p. 1160.
5. American Cancer Society, "Surgery for Breast Cancer," accessed June 2011.
6. Carolyn M. Kaelin, M.D., M.P.H., Francesca Coltrera, Josie Gardiner, and Joy Prouty, *The Breast Cancer Survivor's Fitness Plan*. New York: McGraw-Hill, 2007, p. 40.
7. The National Cancer Institute, "Less Invasive Lymph Node Surgery Safe for Women with Breast Cancer," (www.cancer.gov/clinicaltrials/results/summary/2010/slnb_alnd1110) accessed July 2011.
8. Kaelin, pp. 43–4.
9. U.S. Department of Labor, "Your Rights after a Mastectomy: Womens' Health and Cancer Rights Act." (www.dol.gov/ebsa/pdf/whcra.pdf) accessed July 2011.
10. Hartocollis, Anemona, 2010. "Before Breast Is Removed, A Discussion on Options." *The New York Times*, August 18. (http://www.nytimes.com/2010/08/19/nyregion/19surgery.html) accessed June 2011.
11. The American Cancer Society, "Breast Reconstruction after Mastectomy, (http://www.cancer.org/cancer/breastcancer/more information/breastreconstructionaftermastectomy/breast-reconstruction-after-mastectomy-types-of-br-recon) accessed, June 2011.

12. American Cancer Society, "Breast Reconstruction after Mastectomy." accessed June 2011.

13. U.S. Food and Drug Administration, "FDA Breast Implant Consumer Handbook: – 2004 – Breast Implant Surgery and Related Issues" http://www.fda.gov/MedicalDevices/ProductsandMedicalProcedures/ImplantsandProsthetics/BreastImplants/ucm064176.htm) accessed June 2011, pp. 57–8.

14. Hartocollis, Anemona, 2010. Before a Breast Is Removed, A Discussion on Options. *The New York Times*, August 18. (http://www.nytimes.com/2010/08/19/nyregion/19surgery.html).

15. The National Cancer Institute, "*BRCA-1 and BRCA-2*: Cancer Risk and Genetic Testing" (http://www.cancer.gov/cancertopics/factsheet/Risk/BRCA) accessed June 2011.

16. Gaylene Bouska Altman, *Delmar's Fundamental and Advanced Nursing Skills*, 2th ed., Clifton Park, NY: Delmar, 2004, p. 692.

17. Altman, 1366.

18. Altman, 897.

19. Altman, 1299–1306.

20. *Stedman's*, 781.

21. *Stedman's*, 863.

22. *Stedman's*, 1754.

23. Hiedi McHugh Pendleton, PhD, OTR/L, FAOTA and Winifrid Schultz-Krohn, PhD, OTR/L, BCP, SWC, FAOTA, Eds., *Pedretti's Occupational Therapy Practice Skills for Physical Dysfunction*, 6th ed., St. Louis, MO: Mosby Elsevier, pp. 1153–4.

24. Hiedi McHugh Pendleton, PhD, OTR/L, FAOTA and Winifrid Schultz-Krohn, PhD, OTR/L, BCP, SWC, FAOTA, Eds., p. 1153.

25. Meyer, Lacey. "Skin Deep, Scars Can Be Managed and Minimized," *Cure Magazine*, Summer 2011, p. 64.

26. Breastcancer.org. "Flap Revisions" (www.breastreconstruction.org/SecondaryProcedures/FlapRevision.html) accessed July 2011.

27. McLaughlin et al., "Prevalence of Lymphedema in Women With Breast Cancer 5 Years After Sentinel Lymph Node Biopsy or Axillary Dissection: Objective Measurements." *Journal of Clinical Oncology*, 2008, 26, 32.

28. Petrek JA, Heleen MC. Incidence of Breast Carcinoma – Related Lymphedema. Cancer 1998; 83:2776–81.

29. Kathryn Schmitz, et al., "Weight Lifting in Women with Breast-Cancer–Related Lymphedema," *New England Journal of Medicine*; 361, 664–73, August 13, 2009.

30. National Lymphedema Network, "Position Statement of the National Lymphedema Network, Topic: Air Travel" (http://www.lymphnet.org/pdfDocs/nlnairtravel.pdf) accessed July 2011.

31. Position Statement of the National Lymphedema Network, Topic: Air Travel.
32. Kaelin, 57–8.
33. U.S. Food and Drug Administration, p. 28.
34. U.S. Food and Drug Administration, pp. 22–3.
35. FDA Website, "Breast Implants: Local Complications and Adverse Outcomes." (www.fda.gov/downloads/MedicalDevices/Productsand-MedicalProcedures/ImplantsandProsthetics/BreastImplants/UCM259 894.pdf) accessed July 2011.
36. Michael D. Stubblefield, M.D., and Christian M. Custudio, M. D., "Upper extremity pain disorder in breast cancer," *Archives of Physical Medicine and Rehabilitiation*, 87, Suppl. 1, March 2006.
37. O.J. Vilhom et al., "The postmastectomy pain syndrome: An epidemiological study on the prevalence of chronic pain after surgery for breast cancer," *The British Journal of Cancer*, 99(4), August 19, 2008.
38. Kathy Steligo, *The Breast Reconstruction Guidebook*, 2nd ed., San Carlos, CA: Carlo Press, 2005, pp. 171–2.
39. Love, 454–5.
40. Step Up, Speak Out, "Axillary Web Syndrome/Cording."
41. Step Up, Speak Out, "Axillary Web Syndrome/Cording."
42. Alexander H. Moskovitz, et al., "Axillary web syndrome after axillary dissection." *The American Journal of Surgery*, 181(5), 434–9, May 2001.
43. Step Up, Speak Out, "Axillary Web Syndrome/Cording."
44. Breastcancer.org, "Delayed Wound Healing," (http://www.breast-cancer.org/treatment/side_effects/wound_healing.jsp) accessed June 2011.

Resources

Breast Cancer General Resources and Support
- *Dr. Susan Love's Breast Book*, 5th edition by Susan M. Love, MD, with Karen Lindsey, Da Capo Press, 2010.
- The American Cancer Society (http://www.cancer.org/)
- Be Bright Pink (http://www.bebrightpink.org/)
- Breastcancer.org website (http://www.breastcancer.org/)
- Cancer Support Community (http://www.cancersupport community.org)
- Livestrong (www.livestrong.org)
- The National Cancer Institute website (http://www.cancer.gov)
- Susan G. Komen website (ww5.komen.org/)
- Young Survivor Coalition (http://www.youngsurvival.org/)
- Support Connection: Breast and Ovarian Cancer Support; Toll Free Hotline: 1-800-532-4290 (http://www.supportconnection.org/)

Breast Implant Safety
- U.S. Food and Drug Administration (http://www.fda.gov/)

Breast Reconstruction and Related Issues
- *The Breast Reconstruction Guidebook*, 2nd edition by Kathy Steligo, Carlo Press, 2005.
- *The Breast Cancer Survivor's Fitness Plan*, by Carolyn M. Kaelin, MD, MPH, McGraw-Hill, 2007.
- Breastreconstruction.org (www.breastreconstruction.org/)

- Breast Reconstruction Matters (www.breastreconstruction matters.com/)
- Breastfree.org (www.breastfree.org/)

Dating and Intimacy after Mastectomy
- *Intimacy After Breast Cancer, Dealing With Your Body, Relationships, and Sex* by Gina Maisano, Square One Publishers, 2010.
- *100 Questions and Answers About Breast Cancer, Sensuality, Sexuality, and Intimacy* by Michael L. Krychman, MD, Susan Kellogg Spadt, PhD, CRNP, and Sandra Finestone, PsyD, Jones and Bartlett Publishers, 2011.

Hereditary Breast Cancer
- Facing Our Risk of Cancer Empowered (www.facingourrisk.org)

Lymphedema Education
- National Lymphedema Network (www.lymphnet.org/)
- Step Up- Speak Out (www.stepup-speakout.org/)

Women's Health and Cancer Rights Act (WHCRA)
- U.S. Department of Labor (www.dol.gov/dol/topic/health-plans/womens.htm)

Finding Credentialed Experts in Your Area

Certified Mastectomy Fitters
- American Board for Certification in Orthotics, Prosthetics, and Pedorthics (www.abcop.org/Pages/Directory.aspx?searchtype=Individual)

Genetic Counselors
- National Society of Genetic Counselors (www.nsgc.org/FindaGeneticCounselor)

Lymphedema Certified Therapists
- Lymphology Association of North America (www.clt-lana.org/)
- National Lymphedema Network (www.lymphnet.org/)

Mental Health
- American Psychosocial Oncology Association (www.apos-society.org)

Index